There were two epidemics in New York City in the dry, hot summer of 1999.

Birds and people were getting sick.

Some were dying.

It took nearly two months to realize that they were different manifestations of the same disease, and that it was caused by an infection never before encountered in the Western Hemisphere—the West Nile virus.

What does it mean when a new infectious disease comes to town?

What were the circumstances that made Staten Island the virus's epicenter of human infections in 2000?

What will be the long term effects of WNV on wildlife?

www.westnilestory.com

West Nile Story

Dickson Despommier

Illustrated by Robert J. Demarest

APPLE TREES PRODUCTIONS, LLC
P.O. BOX 280
NEW YORK, NY 10032

Production and design by Robert J. Demarest and Ramona I. Polvere

Library of Congress Card Number: 00-193572
ISBN 0-9700027-1-8

Manufactured in the United States of America

To all those who dedicate their lives helping to alleviate suffering inflicted on the human condition by emerging infections.

Acknowledgements

Writing a book is a complex process involving the expenditure of large quantities of one's time and energy. However, no matter how diligently one tries to succeed, neither of these elements guarantees a high quality product. It is often the reviewers of its contents and their constructive criticisms and insightful suggestions that elevates it from ordinary prose to clear exposition. I am grateful to the following for reviewing my manuscript and gently reminding me not to change tenses in mid-stream, to avoid cliches like the plague (hmmmm), and to remember to focus the text on my audience, the general reading public. I have not intended this to be a specialty book on some esoteric piece of science. Rather, *West Nile Story* is more of a documentary that anyone could refer to when and if the virus visits his or her neighborhood. In this regard, I am extremely grateful to Marlene Bloom for her careful editing and re-editing of the manuscript, and for her many useful additions and subtractions from it. My only concern now is that I have accumulated a drawer full of omitted thuses, thens, therefores, and hences, with no other apparent usefulness than to remind me not to use them in subsequent writing efforts. A special thanks to two of my microbiology colleagues and good friends, Drs. Vincent Racaniello and Hamish Young for lending their expertise as world-renowned virologists to this project insuring the accuracy of the science behind the words. Similarly, I am very grateful to my good friend and colleague Dr. Robert Gwadz of the National Institutes of Health and to Dr. Frank Collins at the University of Notre Dame for helping to insure that the description of the mosquito biology reflects the current state of knowledge regarding these dangerous creatures. Thank you, Dr. Deborah Nicolls for helping me accumulate, and then interpret the medical and ecological literature that enabled me to piece together large parts of the *West Nile Story*. Without your perseverance and dedication, I would not have been able to proceed. I thank Drs. Charles Knirsch and Josh Stillman for their many useful comments on the manuscript during its early iterations. Without their input, it would not reflect current medical opinion regarding the clinical aspects of the West Nile virus. All of this hopefully has been accomplished without the use of tiresome, undecipherable jargon. I am grateful to Robert Demarest for his input in the design of this book, for illustrating the cover, and for his remarkable, creative sketches used throughout the text to enhance its artistic presentation. Thank you also for your sage advice during our many discussions as to how we might proceed in the market place. I thank Alice Demarest and Judy Sulzberger for encouraging me to finish the job. Thank you Pat Moakley for being there when we were considering seeking outside publishers. Your knowledge of the printing and publishing industries gave us the confidence to proceed as an independent publisher. Finally, thank you Ramona Polvere for being the hands and the brains behind the computer, and for creatively incorporating all of our disparate design ideas into a coherent, seamless document.

West Nile Story

Table of Contents

Chapter 1. The Mysterious Stranger

Chapter 2. No Rain, Dead Birds

Chapter 3. Who Done It And How (Maybe)

Chapter 4. Patterns of Nature:
It's Déjà Vu Over And Over Again

Chapter 5. Is Anybody Out There?

Chapter 6. Mosquitoes: Natural Born Killers

Chapter 7. Viruses Rule

Epilogue

Literature on the West Nile Virus

Index

The Mysterious Stranger

St. Louis Blues

Six people were admitted to Flushing Hospital in Queens, New York between August 12 and August 23, 1999, with similar enough symptoms of high fever, altered mental status, and headache to make it probable that they were suffering from the same thing. The fact that they all came from northern Queens made it even more probable. But suffering from what?

A routine culture screen for a few suspected bacterial or fungal microbes was negative, although that wasn't surprising since the growing suspicion was that these patients were experiencing an encephalitis-like disease, probably of viral origin. The culture tests run in the hospital diagnostic microbiology laboratory could not detect viral infections.

In order to do so would have required inoculating serum and cerebrospinal fluid samples into tissue culture. This method for viral diagnosis is not routinely carried out at most hospital facilities, including the one in Flushing.

As the illness progressed, it became more and more apparent that viral encephalitis was the correct diagnosis. Within three weeks of admission, three elderly patients had died of the suspected illness.

These findings gave notice to the rest of New York City that something serious was in progress. On August 23, Dr. Deborah Asnis of Flushing Hospital notified Dr. Marci Layton of the New York City Department of Health (NYCDOH) of these early cases, and Dr. Layton contacted the Centers for Disease Control and Prevention (CDC) in Atlanta, Georgia for assistance in an encephalitis outbreak of unknown origin. The CDC was always on the alert to respond to calls such as this.

As a first step in the process to identify the cause(s) of illness, the CDC sent Dr. Asnis' samples of blood and cerebrospinal fluid collected from each patient, along with brain tissues from the three deceased victims to Dr. Duane Gubler, director of the Division of Vector-borne Diseases Laboratory at the branch of the CDC in Fort Collins, Colorado. The answer came back quickly. It was probably caused by a single agent, St. Louis encephalitis virus (SLE). The diagnosis was based on an antibody reaction routinely used in their laboratory to identify that encephalitis causing virus. As good and reliable as that test was, it was not specific enough to distinguish among viruses causing encephalitis in the United States and those found elsewhere.

To confound things even more, the Queens serum samples gave a positive but weak reaction, to which the closest match was the St. Louis encephalitis virus. The Fort Collins serologists concluded that it must be SLE, since it was the most likely choice. They might have reasoned that the lack of a strong positive reaction probably related to the specific (new?) strain of SLE involved in the outbreak. A slight difference in protein structure of the viral particles could result in a weakened intensity of the interaction of antibodies with the virus without changing the diagnosis. That they failed to test the sera against the West Nile virus (WNV) was natural enough, considering that the WNV agent had never before been encountered in the western hemisphere. Therefore, even though the CDC had all the proper reagents and the capability to detect it, the test was never run.

The West Nile virus is related to SLE, and they both constitute part of a larger family of genetically related viruses called flaviviruses. The prefix "flavi" means yellow, since one of its more notorious members is the yellow fever virus. Flaviviruses have at least one thing in common, something referred to in the jargon of microbiologists as a "cross reacting" protein. This allows the serologist to identify, at a first level, whether or not an unknown virus is a member of this group by using an antibody made against these generic proteins. To distinguish individual family members often requires a more sophisticated approach, in which the genetic material of the virus is compared using computer-assisted programs. The latter strategy was not employed by the CDC prior to their announcement that the Queens victims most probably succumbed to a new strain of SLE.

The Sound Of Zebras

A commonly held adage among pathologists in the United States that has been adopted by many other health professionals as their credo when they encounter the unknown or unfamiliar is: "When you hear hoof beats think horses, not zebras." In other words, start solving a problem by considering the most likely scenarios first before moving on to more exotic possibilities. It's the familiar that greatly influences the initial attempt to explain a given finding. Of course, pathologists in Africa hear the sound of zebras, not horses.

Location, Location, Location

St. Louis encephalitis infections had occurred before in New York State, but never in New York City. Even though it was unusual, finding it there did not seem entirely out of the realm of possibility. Again, the most reasonable explanation for the cause of the encephalitis outbreak seemed to lie in the positive, albeit weak, antibody reaction to the St. Louis encephalitis virus. The physicians at Flushing Hospital were notified of the findings, and all personnel involved with the epidemic at the NYCDOH and CDC went about the job of determining how many other cases of SLE there were throughout the New York area. Since the virus is transmitted to humans by the bite of infected mosquitoes, it was reasoned that it was probably in other places, as well. In retrospect, the hoof beats were from zebras.

Kicking It Up A Notch

By the 6th of September, things began to escalate on all fronts. There were now five confirmed cases, as many as 34 others awaiting final diagnosis, and the first two deaths. Although hundreds of native bird deaths had been recorded throughout the city starting in late July, it wasn't until September 9, that exotic birds began dying at the Bronx Zoo. Dr. Tracy McNamara, a pathologist there, became involved in the unfolding drama surrounding one of the world's great metropolitan communities. After autopsying all birds that died inside the zoo exhibits, and some that had died outside the zoo, as well, she was no closer to explaining their deaths than before the investigation began. McNamara suspected, based on the similarity of their presenting pathological conditions, that they had all been felled by the same disease, whatever it was. Therefore, no one working either from the human side or the wildlife side made the connection between the twin epidemics. More zebras.

The next day, another human case was confirmed, and the number of suspected cases rose to 48. This was now more than a worrisome local health problem in Queens. The same evening, specially equipped helicopters hovered above major highways and residential areas deemed most at risk from invasion by mosquitoes, and sprayed misty clouds of insecticide (malathion and pyrethriods) in their wake. A general health warning was issued by Dr. Neal Cohen, Commissioner of the NYCDOH, about how to avoid contact with both mosquitoes and the insecticides.

Three days later, on the 13th, 11 confirmed cases, 3 deaths, and a total of 65 probable cases had been identified. Nearly all of them were over the age of 50. Numerous reports of new dead bird sightings filled the headlines of the local and national news, as the infection cast its shadow over a wider and wider range of hosts and territory.

Some mosquitoes collected from Connecticut tested positive. By combining small samples of the same species of adult mosquito into "pools," then analyzing each pool for virus, virologists, using the same test as employed by the CDC, showed that *Culex pipiens* and *Aedes vexan* harbored the St. Louis virus particles.

At about this same time, a few horses on Long Island died of an illness presumed to be this new variety of SLE, causing further confusion and deepening the mystery.

Meanwhile, on the 20th of September, the CDC took another long look at all their test results and began to suspect that it was not St. Louis encephalitis, after all. The same day, the CDC laboratories in Fort Collins received additional specimens from the scene of the outbreak; this time it was tissue samples from dead birds (crows and exotic birds from the epidemic at the Bronx Zoo) sent to them by Dr. Beverly Schmitt, chief veterinary medical officer, Diagnostic Virology Laboratory at the National Veterinary Services Laboratories in Ames, Iowa.

Don't Look Now, But...

On the 21st, Leonard Spano, County Clerk for Westchester County, New York, announced that two confirmed and one probable case of SLE had occurred there, as well. Finding more dead crows in the same county reinforced the urgent need to identify what it was that was rapidly spreading out from its epicenter in the Fort Totten area of northern Queens. Mr. Spano also conceded that spraying by helicopter was not an option, but rather a necessity if the county was to have any chance at all of containing the mosquitoes responsible for dissemination of the virus. In contrast to New York City, Mr. Spano elected to spray only pyrethriods, not malathion, as it was judged by his health commissioner, Dr. Joshua Lipsman, that the latter was too toxic for general use.

More dead crows, some found in Westport, Connecticut, tested positive for SLE. Despite these futile attempts at controlling the vectors, an ecological network of infection was rapidly and inexorably being established by the virus in the northeastern part of the United States.

The CDC conducted additional tests on the brain tissues of deceased victims to look for the virus, itself. Dr. Sharif Zaki and his team employed an antibody test designed to detect the common protein shared by all flavivirus members. Their results were positive, revealing the presence of the virus family member protein in the brain tissue sections. This important finding encouraged investigators to proceed further to attempt to isolate and study the virus directly from these human tissue samples

While all this activity was going forward, on September 21, Dr. Ian Lipkin, director of the Emerging Infections Laboratory of the University of California, Irvine, was invited to join in the hunt by Drs. Leo Grady and Cinnia Huang of the Griffin Laboratory for Virological Studies at the New York State Department of Health in Albany. Realizing that data of a more specific nature were needed to finally identify which virus was causing the epidemic, Drs. Grady and Huang called in outside assistance.

The Griffin Laboratory had fallen on hard times due mostly to attrition and lack of sustained financial support. The viruses the lab could test for were limited to those known to occur within the United States. Grady and Huang submitted five brain samples from autopsies to Dr. Lipkin's laboratory for further analysis. Lipkin's laboratory is, in his own words, "...dedicated to the identification and characterization of infectious agents using molecular biological methods."

The same day, Dr. Lipkin's team began the work of sequencing the viral RNA genome. Remarkably, by the next day, they had identified a portion of the genome of the flavivirus in three of the brain samples as being related to the West Nile virus, and the day after, September 23, had extracted the complete length of the virus's single stranded RNA molecule, and cloned it. Lipkin's preliminary results were immediately e-mailed to a special internet site, ProMED (program for monitoring emerging diseases), a "chat room" for the exchange of preliminary data and ideas regarding epidemics occurring anywhere in the world. It is avidly read on a daily basis by most scientists who specialize in infectious diseases.

Sequencing the cloned molecule, now converted to a more usable form (DNA) began that day, and ultimately led to the identification of the specific virus responsible for the health problems in Queens. The work was finished in just a little over 24 hours, an accomplishment worthy of praise even in the most sophisticated scientific circles, considering the source of the starting material.

Dr. Vincent Deubel of the Pasteur Institute in Paris, read of Dr. Lipkin's findings on ProMED and immediately made available to him sequences of cloned genomes Deubel's laboratory had collected from a variety of West Nile virus outbreaks in Romania, Egypt, Israel, Italy, and South Africa, among others. The genomic sequence that Dr. Lipkin's group had determined from the virus in the brain samples from the victims of Queens, matched exactly with the strain that caused an epidemic in Israel in 1998—and with no other.

On the 24th of September, Dr. Lipkin informed the New York State Department of Health and Dr. Steven Ostroff, the CDC epidemiology officer in charge of the epidemic, that his group had determined the complete viral genome sequence. The California team got it right, correctly identifying the causative agent of the encephalitis epidemic as none other than the West Nile virus. Announcements from New York City, New York State, and the CDC to a beleaguered public followed shortly, eliciting more questions than answers about the events of that most trying summer in The Big Apple.

Tempest In A Teapot

Hurricane Floyd had passed through on September 16, breaking the weather conditions which favored the spread of the virus to humans. The epidemic was waning. No new cases were reported after October 16. In all, a total of 62 clinical cases and seven deaths had occurred. One was a very unlucky Canadian citizen who had briefly visited the New York area, only to die of the infection shortly after returning to his home in Toronto. The tumult on the human side of the epidemic finally stopped and it was time to reflect.

What had really happened in Queens and the rest of the metropolitan area? If all the details of the epidemic were known, could anything be done to prevent it from happening again? Will the wildlife that somehow evaded the infection this time succumb to it in subsequent years? Can a vaccine be produced in time to prevent infection in horses and other domestic animals?

Chapter 2

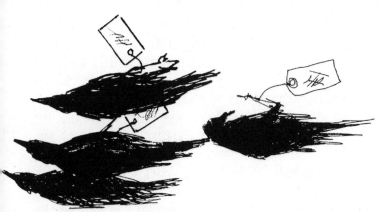

No Rain, Dead Birds

We're Having A Heat Wave

Around the country, droughts and off-the-scale temperatures dominated the local and national news, with Cincinnati and Houston catching most of the headlines. Both cities had recorded many days of temperatures above 100° F, and Houston had more than a week of 105+F degree days. The heat was devastating to wildlife, and became life-threatening for humans, too. In fact, many elderly and some very young people died as the result of inadequate protection from the heat. Dehydration was the main cause, but in some cases, a core body temperature exceeding 106° F was recorded just prior to death.

Back east, the situation was just as desperate. On May 24, 1999, the National Weather Service station in New York City's Central Park registered 1.24 inches of precipitation in its rain gauges. Rainfall that month had been somewhat below average, with a total of 3.74 inches. Nothing to worry about, though; the upstate reservoirs which New York City uses to slake its gotham-sized thirst (1.3 billion gallons/day) were at near full capacity (about 550 billion gallons), and the outlook for the coming summer was generally upbeat. The Dow and the NASDAQ were up (well, mostly), good beach weather was just around the corner, the 33 outdoor municipal pools (and numerous mini-pools) scattered throughout the five boroughs would open in June, and the handful of small farms still operating in the southern tier of the state were doing reasonably well at the start of the growing season. All in all, the city appeared to be headed for a normal summer.

But the only constant thing about nature is that it keeps changing. Over the next 35 days, virtually no precipitation in any form fell to the ground, and on June 29, only 0.19 inches of rain hit the parched sidewalks of a city reluctantly settling into the grips of another drought.

In the Northeast, the 1980s were typified by yearly droughts, both in the winter and summer, but in the last few years rainfall had been normal. New Yorkers were getting used to the idea that extended dry periods may not be a permanent fixture of their summers, when the rains again failed to materialize. This drought extended throughout July; only 0.44 inches fell for the entire month. In August, just over 1.3 inches of rain was scattered over a period of 25 days, making the summer of '99 one of the driest ever recorded for the region. The weather broke temporarily on August 26, when 1.58 inches was recorded in the rain gauge in Central Park over a 24-hour period. Most of it disappeared into the ground faster than a New York minute. The hydrological cycle had been partially restored, at least for the moment. This rain event, and Hurricane Floyd that followed the next month, most likely enabled a population of mosquitoes to establish the West Nile virus firmly in this hemisphere.

Fun In The Sun

It wasn't just the lack of rain that made life uncomfortable. The heat associated with the drought placed added pressure on New Yorkers to seek out relief wherever they could find it. Many thousands left the area, opting for traditional pilgrimages to vacation spots outside the city. For most who had to stay and work, air conditioning solved the problem indoors, but going outside for any reason during daylight hours was often hellish.

During the last week in June, after the city schools had let out for the summer, the municipal pools finally opened. Kids and adults by the hundreds of thousands descended on them like so many wildebeest seeking out the last waterhole on a drought-stricken savanna. For those who could not find their way to a pool, the fire hydrants, with and without restrictors, served as substitutes. These convenient fountains were treasured oases, spraying relief onto groups of urban bathers, with an occasional "spritz" or two onto passing vehicles. Unsuspecting drivers (usually from out of state) with their windows down got the outsides and part of the insides of their cars washed, free of charge, by local curbside "car wash" experts. People went to the beaches, where sea breezes offered them some degree of comfort.

Some residents of Queens, particularly those living in the northern sections, had other choices for avoiding the heat. Over 150 private pools dot the borough's backyard landscape of single family houses and garden apartments. Most are above-ground structures that offer their owners a certain privacy when compared to the municipal pool system. Many are shared on a daily basis with extended family and close neighbors, so pool-side picnics and barbecues become treasured summer events during most normal years. But this was not a normal year. While June temperatures had been about normal with just six days in the 90's, July was another story, with 15 days soaring above 90° F, and three exceeding 100° F. This, too, would prove an important ecological factor for establishing and maintaining the epidemic.

In early July, the alert to conserve water was issued from the city's Department of Environmental Conservation. Washing cars and watering lawns was openly discouraged by the city. Automobiles became dusty, and many, but not all, lawns turned brown. Some owners of backyard pools cut back on their use, voluntarily complying with the water alert. In addition, the rising energy costs associated with high electricity demand (running of air conditioners, etc), forced frugal pool owners to turn off filtering pumps and other pool-related gadgets.

Many owners went on vacations for extended periods. The chlorine in their unused pools evaporated, turning them into mini-reservoirs of stagnant, warm water—the perfect breeding habitat for some mosquito species. The ramifications of this single act of benign neglect were to become evident throughout the neighborhood.

In The Cool, Cool, Cool Of The Evening

Other residents of Queens lived next to those who went away, and kept their pools filled and well-maintained as the drought deepened. Parties were planned. The summer was finally here, and there were steaks to be grilled, racks of baby back ribs to be slowly turned and carefully brushed with special home-made sauces, and jokes and stories to be shared over ice cold pitchers of tea and tall glasses generously filled and re-filled with gin and tonic water.

Citronella candles blazed on into the night, as the weekend gatherings continued throughout the hot summer, with guests no doubt doing what guests do best when offered the opportunity to indulge themselves in a cool, comfortable place. They lingered into the morning hours, laughing, drinking, and eating their way through the weekends.

Typical for all droughts, no matter where they occur, nearly all bird species had long gone from the area, driven away by the heat and dry conditions. Without birds to feed on, but with new breeding sites to use, *Culex pipiens* switched to humans for their blood meals. These polluted water-loving mosquitoes survived the dry heat of the dog days of August and were able to take full advantage of the situation, enjoying a nightly feast of their own! Of particular significance to that borough of New York City, of the approximately two million people who live in Queens, well over 400,000 are over the age of 60. These individuals were the ones most susceptible to the lethal effects of the virus once it gained access to their neighborhoods.

The Urban Wildlife Scene

In Manhattan, museum and hotel fountains stopped their rhythmic dances, and the soothing noises made by sheets of water cascading down the granite walls of pocket parks were replaced by the sound of silence. Birds gathered near the reservoir in Central Park for a drink, but the ingredients for their picnics—seeds, insects, and worms—had become scarce due to the dry weather. They had a better chance finding these food items in areas that were still thriving, despite the droughty conditions: the edges of ponds, riverbanks, and the parts of urban forests that bordered them. Back yards in the outlying boroughs that had not been watered in weeks were practically barren, and were by-passed in favor of greener pastures.

Large numbers of these displaced birds found refuge near the Bronx Zoo, which had a special dispensation from the water alert due to the requirements of its permanent residents. Its numerous duck ponds and wading pools still allowed exotic birds of all feathers to attract the attention of the growing hordes of visitors. The Congo gorilla forest habitat exhibit commemorating the 100th anniversary of the zoo had opened on June 24 to well-deserved rave reviews, and it attracted overflow crowds of visitors each day for several months thereafter.

The Bronx River meanders next to the zoo complex, fed in part by the outlets from the zoo ponds. It acted like a magnet for the displaced birds;

they were drawn to it from the now dry and lifeless surrounding landscape. Adjacent to the zoo complex, the banks of the Bronx River are shaded by 40 acres of native forest, a portion of which still lies within the Bronx Botanical Gardens, proper. Inside the gardens, the forest has never been clear cut. In the early part of the 1700s, this stand of trees was referred to as The Hemlock Grove. According to Todd Forrest, curator of woody plants at the Bronx Botanical Gardens, the hemlocks had disappeared from that area, succumbing to woolly adelgid, a disease caused by a beetle (*Adelges tsugae*) thought to originate in Asia. It has been in the United States since 1924. Over time, this small patch of nature has evolved into a climax forest of oak, tulip, and maple. A few remaining hardwood trees there are well over 300 years old.

The river and its banks are alive with remnant assemblages of fauna and flora that have been pushed and shoved into this small zone by relentless encroachment from all directions. New York City has nearly 4,000 acres of intact forested area within its five boroughs; a small miracle considering the fact that over nine million people live practically on top of them.

Dead Birds

In late July, in a seemingly unrelated event to the West Nile episode, 87 birds of many kinds were found dead in one small patch of Central Park. Analysis showed that they had all died as the result of ingesting the highly toxic insecticide, carbofuran. At the same time, the tissues of dead birds found in other city parks were shown also to contain this poison. What had happened that had caused these unfortunate deaths was never determined, but a deliberate poisoning event is hard to argue against, considering that all the parks were involved. The New York chapter of the Audubon Society surely believed that was the case.

In insects, carbofuran is a potent inhibitor of the nervous system, preventing it from transmitting signals to other parts of the arthropod's body. Death comes quickly and decisively as the result of even a single exposure. A bird's nervous system is equally sensitive to that toxin.

The chemical comes in the form of tiny white pellets that birds and other animals mistake for bits of food. It is a favorite among private exterminators, but its not used much by the city health department. A demented person with a Tom Lehrer complex may well have been responsible for that dastardly deed, since the overall pattern of bird deaths obviously did not fit the description of an accidental spill. Regardless of who caused it, the poisonings were not without significance when placed into the context of the West Nile virus outbreak.

Red Herring

During early and mid-August, an increasing number of dead birds, especially crows, were discovered throughout the metropolitan area. It seemed reasonable to attribute their deaths to the ingestion of carbofuran. One interviewee on a local news program even went so far as to venture that the drought itself may have caused some of the bird deaths, though how this could happen is not obvious given the fact that birds can detect and then fly at will to any available aquatic environment.

By late August, it was becoming more and more apparent that poisoning was not the cause of the problem. A retrospective study on re-tested birds collected at various times throughout the summer revealed that at least one crow had died of West Nile virus on August 9. It was also noted throughout the epidemic by a few of those who found some affected birds still alive, that the victims seemed to die more slowly than would have been expected from poisoning. Rather, the birds behaved as if they had been injured or infected with a lethal microbe. This clue was essentially ignored, explained away as either a variation in the age of the birds affected, or something to do with their food supply. Every guess turned out to be wrong.

Are We There Yet?

The mystery deepened when the epidemic visited the zoo. From August 10 through September 23, scores of native birds of all types were found stiff-legged on the grounds surrounding the Bronx Zoo. On September 9, exotic birds on display at the zoo began dying (five Chilean Flamingos, several Bald Eagles, Guanary Cormorants, Bronze-winged Ducks, Black-billed Magpies, Snowy Owls, and many others). All appeared to have died from the same disease, although what had caused their deaths was not obvious, even after the autopsies were performed. This unsettling event triggered a red alert and the hunt for the causes of all bird deaths throughout the city went into maximum warp drive. It is interesting to note that none of the exotic bird deaths occurred among species originating from either Africa, the Middle East, or Europe. Birds that had died outside the zoo, aside from the incidents in the parks, tested negative for carbofuran poisoning, and exhibited no signs of dehydration, leaving the cause of death for all bird species up in the air.

For The Birds

Dr. Ward Stone is a widely respected wildlife pathologist who works for the State of New York and had been hard at work on this intractable problem for more than a month. He was the one responsible for the discovery that birds in the parks had died of carbofuran poisoning.

In late August, he, along with everyone else, learned through a news release from the New York City Department of Health about an outbreak of St. Louis encephalitis (SLE) among a few residents of northern Queens. When questioned about the possibility that the birds might also be dying from SLE, he explained that this could not happen after infection with that particular virus, since no bird species native to the United States has ever died from SLE. He further explained that North American birds are highly adapted to it, serving as a reservoir, giving it to mosquitoes that then occasionally bite people. Humans can become sick, exhibiting all the signs and symptoms of encephalitis, but even they rarely die as the result of the infection. According to the Centers for Disease Control and Prevention, a total of nine isolated cases of St. Louis encephalitis virus had occurred in upstate New York, and these were spread out over a 34-year period from 1964 to 1998. But it came as only a small surprise to health officials that this virus, known to occur occasionally in New York State, was now in New York City, as well.

Culture Club

Meanwhile, back at the Bronx Zoo, Dr. Tracy McNamara, an avian pathologist and senior member of the support staff responsible for maintaining the health of the animals at the zoo, and her colleagues, had now become deeply involved in the bird epidemic. Autopsies of all the exotic bird victims revealed a similar pattern of disease, but there was not enough evidence to make a definitive diagnosis. Samples of all their tissues were immediately collected, frozen, and sent to Dr. Beverly Schmitt at the U.S. Department of Agriculture National Veterinary Services Laboratories in Ames, Iowa.

Dr. Schmitt also received tissues from crows that had died in another part of New York City. She and her co-workers began a carefully planned, systematic search and analysis for all kinds of infectious agents. They inoculated small, homogenized samples of the bird tissues into bacterial culture tubes containing a variety of growth media, and into tissue culture dishes to detect the growth of any viruses that might be present. The samples were incubated at various temperatures, and the scientists waited for the results. What they were hoping for in the search for viruses was the death of any of the cells that grew as a single, contiguous layer over the entire surface of the culture plate. Abnormalities of the cellular layer (holes in the layer or distorted cells) would mean that a virus was present in the bird tissues, and that each viral particle inoculated into the dish had infected an individual cell. Over a 24-48 hour period, the virus would have replicated, making changes in the cell layer apparent when viewed under the microscope.

Within days, they found what they were looking for—cell pathology—but the follow-up experiment gave a somewhat disappointing, non-specific result. They had successfully determined that all the birds were infected with a single species of virus, but its identity was not apparent even after viewing it under the electron microscope.

Nevertheless, they could discern that it closely resembled those in several related groups; the togaviridae and flaviviridae. Both of these known virus groups are of the same diameter, around 40 nanometers, as were the viruses identified from the zoo and crow isolates. In addition, all shared the same general round shape. However, when new tissue cultures were prepared in which antibodies against all known domestic viruses were included into the growth medium before inoculating the unknown agent into the culture tube, the new virus still infected the cells. In other words, the virus was not prevented from continuing its growth by any of the antibodies made against domestic viruses. This proved that the samples were different from any agent on hand in their laboratory.

As another way of measuring their ability to induce disease, the samples were inoculated into chicken embryos. The results showed that the viruses induced a similar pattern of pathology as seen in the tissue cultures, but gave no further clues as to their true identities.

At that point, Dr. Schmitt deferred to another government facility that had a more complete repertoire of frozen samples of virus and the antibodies against them, the CDC at Fort Collins, Colorado. On September 20, she forwarded all laboratory specimens and resulting culture fluids containing the virus to the CDC, and waited, along with Dr. McNamara's group at the Bronx Zoo, for new results.

The CDC laboratory at Fort Collins is world famous. The vector-borne disease laboratory there is headed by Dr. Duane Gubler, a medical entomologist with an outstanding scientific reputation, and who is internationally renowned. The facility is staffed by a number of highly trained and respected virologists, many of whom are experts in arboviruses (arthopod-borne diseases). It has an extensive repertoire of known viruses that infect humans and a wide variety of animals, including birds, collected over years from around the world. In addition, it has an exhaustive array of anti-sera against most of them, so rapid identification of any viral particle is possible.

After working around the clock for two days, the final diagnosis of West Nile-like virus was made by the CDC lab, giving a more definitive and quite unexpected outcome to the month-and-a-half-long quest. The CDC learned of a significant, related result from another laboratory on September 23, and together with their findings conducted further tests. The next day, the CDC announced they had definitively proven that the bird infections and the people infections were caused by the same agent, the West Nile virus.

Mosquito, Bird, Man

The other result that the CDC had learned about, which helped them finally solve the puzzle came from a totally unexpected source, Dr. Ian Lipkin's virus laboratory at the University of California at Irvine. At about the same time that the bird samples were shipped to Iowa, brain samples from five of the fatalities in Queens were forwarded to Dr. Lipkin by scientists working at the Griffin Laboratory at the New York State Health Department. Lipkin's group proceeded to isolate the virus from the infected tissues, and sequenced its RNA, proving that it was the West Nile virus.

The parallel timelines of the events leading up to the identification of the virus in birds and people now were connected, and both resolved into a single, coherent body of data describing how this newest infectious disease agent of North America behaved during the summer drought of 1999.

By the time the CDC made its historic declaration on September 24, over 1,900 presumed infections had already occurred in Queens, alone. Probably another 2-4,000 human infections occurred in the surrounding communities, but serological surveys were not conducted in any other place to verify this speculation.

When Hurricane Floyd burst onto the scene on September 16, in addition to scattering mosquitoes, birds, and debris in its wake, it also re-arranged the landscape as only hurricanes can do. North Carolina was hardest hit, and is still in recovery from the torrential rains that left more than 20 inches of water on the ground in less than 24 hours. Floyd also heralded the end of the epidemic in humans. By October 16, no more cases occurred, and West Nile was apparently finished for the year. Not so for horses, birds and other wildlife. The epidemic raged on, spreading from New York to Connecticut to Massachusetts, and from northern New Jersey, south to Delaware.

Evolution, Not Revolution

So, what does the future hold in store for the birds and other wildlife regarding this uninvited guest? The carcasses of dead birds will undoubtedly continue to litter the landscape of the northeastern half of the United States as the WNV epidemic reemerges from year to year. Whether it will spread even farther afield (into the midwest or far west) is too difficult to predict without additional years of data collection regarding its movement among the wildlife in this geographic region.

It's reasonable to assume that the majority of birds living in endemic areas will not be bitten by infected mosquitoes. This does not insure that they will not become infected, however, since it has been recently shown that the WNV can be transmitted from crow to crow without the need for an infected mosquito. There are probably some crows and other native bird species, too, that, by chance, have an innate immunity to the virus, even before encountering it. They may survive to carry on, replacing those lost to the epidemic.

To understand the dynamics of WNV transmission and its consequences to our native birds, we need to compare it with the situation that has evolved among the birds and vectors of WNV in its place of origin—Africa. In that continent, no birds die from the infection due to the fact that they have adapted to it over long periods of time.

The relationship between native African birds and some species of European birds, and the WNV represents a balance between the parasite and its hosts. This process usually takes many centuries of repeated exposure to an infectious agent to develop. In contrast, in this country most bird species are highly susceptible to it, since they have had no prior history of association with the WNV. The exceptions are the numerous introduced bird species from Europe and Africa. The genes that control their immune responses enable them to recognize the virus and dampen its effects. This would explain the lack of exotic bird deaths at the Bronx Zoo among those species imported from Africa, Europe, or the Middle East. Starlings, English sparrows, and pigeons are some of the imports derived from European stocks living in the U.S.A. Few if any of these species have died as the result of exposure to the WNV.

Over time, the native birds of North America will undoubtedly adapt to the virus, and perhaps the virus may even "attenuate" or reduce its ability to induce disease, thus resulting in a decrease in its rate of mortality. However, it's hard to say just how much time will be needed for this balance to be achieved. Attenuation can occur by what is known as serial passage, and happens naturally when an infectious agent is transmitted again and again through a given population of host species. Birds adapt by being selected for resistance. As suggested, ones that cannot resist die, leaving behind the small number that can. Over time, again how much time is not known, the resistant birds will restore their numbers and life will go on as before.

Nature Abhors A Vacuum

As we have seen, the introduction of the WNV had widespread negative effects on both wildlife and humans. It is unfortunate that conditions were just right to allow the infection to establish itself and take off. There is no turning back. WNV now is an ensconced member of the New World family of encephalitis viruses, and will undoubtedly cause illness for wild birds, horses and other mammals, including us, when just the right conditions occur. There are also, predictably, newer entities that have not yet made the scene. An open niche is too inviting to nature for her not to fill it with something, no matter that it may cause grief and pain. So goes the natural world, of which we have always been a part, but are only consciously reminded of it at times like these.

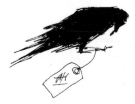

Chapter 3

Who Done It
And How (maybe)

Strangers In A Strange Land

The introduction of any life form into a part of the world that never had it before is known to biologists as bioinvasion. The arrival of a new species into a given environment can have several possible outcomes, not all of which are bad. For example, the species could be excluded by the native assemblages of plants and animals, and never establish itself. This is a good thing. Alternatively, it could just settle itself in among the wildlife and become integrated without too much disturbance. This is usually a good thing, but exceptions abound. Lastly, some introductions can get out of control in their new-found ecosystems, and out-compete established life forms, upsetting native inter-relationships. The last scenario is almost always bad for the local wildlife.

Plants like purple loosestrife, phragmites, and kudzu have established themselves in North America, displacing native plants by their aggressive growth patterns. The Japanese beetle, gypsy moth, German cockroach, Asian tiger mosquito (a potential vector for WNV), pigeon, Norway rat, starling, and English house sparrow are a few of the many animals that have established residence in the U.S.A. without a proper biological passport. Many of these organisms are considered pests by most of us, and are even deemed unwanted guests by the ecologists who study them.

Paradise Lost

Geographic regions that are isolated are particularly susceptible to bioinvasion. The islands of Hawaii, for example, are under constant attack, and their native fauna and flora have suffered much. The introduction of *Culex pipiens* resulted in a "double whammy." The mosquito arrived and immediately made a pest out of itself to the human inhabitants. In addition, these new unwanted arrivals carried bird malaria with them, an often fatal protozoan disease, and unleashed this deadly parasite, causing the extinction of numerous native bird species.

Australia, too, has borne the brunt of introductions of non-native animals and plants such as rabbits, pigs, camels, European trees and shrubs, and other life that have caused permanent changes to the landscape.

The introduction of trout into New Zealand in the late 1800s resulted in the extinction of great numbers of aquatic insects species. Until then, native insects had had no fish predators. Stream insects in river systems with indigenous trout populations crawl under rocks to avoid predation. In contrast, New Zealand species lived on the upper surface of the rocks, exposed to the sun; easy pickings for the newcomers.

In fact, there are very few places on earth that have not had, at some time in their histories, massive invasions of plant and animal species. The radiation of humankind over the surface of the earth during the beginning stages of our own evolution affected more and more of the life that got in the way of our migrations. The extinction of the wooly mammoth, the Dodo bird, the passenger pigeon, and many, many more life forms attests to the efficiency of our ability to affect other wildlife in an adverse way. We still are doing it today. Steamships whose hulls are filled with Norway rats and other vermin dock at every major port city throughout the world. These stowaways have distributed themselves so well that now they constitute essentially a global community of rats, cockroaches, and pigeons. The feral cat and dog are two others that rival the wharf rat for dominance of the back alley ecosystems and garbage heaps of most cities throughout the world.

It should not surprise us to learn that infectious diseases dependent upon vectors follow similar patterns of distribution. If someone harbors an infection and travels into a part of the world that does not have the appropriate vector, there can be no transmission. This applies to most vector-borne infectious tropical diseases. Malaria is a notable exception, since many competent anopheline vector mosquitoes live world-wide, even in temperate zones, and help to maintain its cycle anywhere they are found including here.

A Movable Feast

In the case of WNV, the mosquitoes responsible for transmission among the birds already exist in most parts of the world due to their distribution by international travel. In the United States, they regularly transmit a variety of encephalitis viruses by feeding on both birds and some mammals, including horses and people. Eastern equine, St Louis, La Crosse, and Western equine are encephalitis viruses that fall into this group of domestic woes. Birds distribute the agents throughout their ecological ranges, which can be extensive because of their annual migrations. While some varieties of ticks have also been shown to be capable of transmitting the WNV, most vector experts dismiss this group of arthropods as being unimportant to the epidemiology of both the human and wildlife aspect of the infection.

When the West Nile virus entered our part of the world, our mosquitoes, mostly *Culex pipiens*, *C. restuans*, and *Aedes japonicus*, were happy to oblige, and gave it to scads of new hosts.

The West Nile Express

All of this information may be interesting, but the crucial question is: How did the WNV actually get here? To attempt to answer, we are forced to hypothesize about the events that might have led to its introduction. Recall that the genomic sequence of the strain of WNV in the U.S.A. matched identically with only one other, and that one was isolated in 1998 from an Israeli-raised domestic goose during the outbreak in that country. The other 22 strains meticulously maintained by Dr. Deubel at the Pasteur Institute in Paris did not even come close to matching with ours. The next closest one, from Romania, was only 97% identical.

Recall also that the climatic conditions that prevailed in New York during the summer of 1999 were unusually hot and very dry, the very same environmental conditions that spawned previous outbreaks across most parts of Africa, the Middle East, and throughout the Mediterranean basin of Europe. More on this aspect later.

So now we are ready to put all the facts together and to make some sense out of what happened to initiate, maintain, and finally to end the epidemic. What follows is speculation, but speculation based on a host of solid facts.

The medical ecology of WNV on Israeli goose farms may go a long way towards explaining how the whole thing got started on our side of the Atlantic.

In the Middle East, *Culex univittatus* and *C. molestus* are the dominant vector mosquito species for WNV. They are closely related in both their feeding preferences and breeding site selections to *Culex pipiens*. They feed on birds when they are available and over-winter as adults. Both species also like to breed in stagnant, polluted water, which makes them the ideal kind of insects for living near humans in that arid region of the world. Geese need a constant source of water, and mosquitoes can and often do breed in these farm-created habitats. It is not too difficult to imagine how a young Israeli farm worker or a visitor to a goose farm might have become involved in the epidemic.

Mother Goose Tales

The farm worker or visitor would most likely have been someone who came into close association with the geese. He or she would also have had to schedule a trip to New York, and several days before departure, would have had to be bitten by an infected *Culex univittatus* or *C. molestus* mosquito. Since the incubation period (the time it takes the virus to cause illness after being acquired) for WNV varies somewhat among the strains, 5-10 days would have been a reasonable length of time to allow for the fateful encounter with the mosquito before the trip. This person would most likely have been young, perhaps 5-35 years of age; people who fall within this age group are not usually susceptible to the major pathological effects of the virus, and most will tolerate its presence quite well. Mild fever is usually the only consequence of infection in this age group. In support of this contention, recall that some 1,900 people were estimated to have become infected with the virus in New York and environs in 1999, yet only a handful of them became ill enough to seek medical assistance.

In late July, the traveler got on an airplane and flew to New York. It is estimated that over 300,000 people arrive in New York City from Tel Aviv alone, each month during the height of the summer. Surely one of them could have visited or even worked on a goose farm prior to his or her arrival here in the U.S.

Other theories are less plausible, at least in the opinion of this author and Drs. Vincent Deubel and Ian Lipkin, both of whom acknowledge that a tourist or traveler from Israel to the U.S. could well have "done it."

All other scenarios—European or African birds blown off course during their migration, or illegally imported animals infected with the virus—have a much lower probability. Infected mosquito stowaways could have done it, but getting them to the epicenter of northern Queens or the Bronx Zoo from any airport in the New York metropolitan area is the main problem with this hypothesis. But let's not discount them, altogether. The ways of nature seem rather far-fetched to us until they are revealed, usually by hard-won research efforts. Some of the ways that plants and animals are distributed throughout the world involve such unlikely mechanisms as clinging to birds' feet or being carried long distances (sometimes thousands of miles) by the wind.

The viremia (a term referring to the number of virus particles actually circulating throughout the victim's bloodstream) in our traveler would have had to be high enough for that individual to be able to transmit it to an American *Culex pipiens*. We know that's also an entirely reasonable expectation with this member of the flavivirus family, especially if the infection occurs in a young person. This mode of transmission (endemic) occurs regularly in northern South Africa and southern Egypt.

Upon arrival, the visitor (still viremic) probably joined relatives or friends in northern Queens, where the virus could have easily been picked up by *C. pipiens* breeding in the polluted, warm, standing water of an unused backyard pool. Fort Totten, Queens, was the place from which a crow that had died of the disease was first recovered.

Perhaps our visitor went to the Bronx Zoo, passing the infection on to the local *Aedes japon-*

icus mosquito population, a day feeder, who then would have had the opportunity to pass it on to a few birds and people. These infected birds could then serve as a source of WNV for the local *C. pipiens*. Undoubtedly, the virus amplified maximally inside each infected insect due to the hot weather. These highly viremic mosquitoes in turn, passed it on to their offspring and many more birds, both outside and inside the zoo grounds, and possibly to people visiting there, as well.

Note In Added Proof

As further support for the hypothesis that someone from Israel might have inadvertently introduced WNV into the western hemisphere, in August through September 2000, another WNV outbreak occurred there. Two hundred thirty seven cases were recorded, with 17 deaths. Thousands more were undoubtedly infected. Early migration of African bird species coming down to that region from the Crimea and other breeding sites in Asia, together with an unusually dry, hot summer, combined to create conditions that favored the start of the epidemic.

According to meterologists in Tel Aviv, their summer was one of the driest on record even for that part of the Middle East, supporting the contention that major outbreaks of WNV mainly occur under these conditions.

You Give Me Fever

The epidemic was now on, smoldering among the birds and people throughout the early part of August, completely undetected. People in other parts of the New York area also became infected with the virus. It is possible that these people visited the zoo at just the wrong moment, and became involved in the spreading epidemic. Or perhaps they, too, attended pool parties in Queens.

If this is the way it began, could anything have been done to prevent the introduction of WNV into the United States? Most certainly not, given the unusual conditions needed to establish it here. We were just plain unlucky, and we can be unlucky, again. We can experience an epidemic when conditions favor transmission to us. If a change in the environment brings about rearrangements in the proportions of the normal equation and depletes food supplies of native birds, *Culex pipiens* and other members of this mosquito family will be forced to forage on humans.

"...and Staten Island, too."

In the Northeast, a total of 20 people became ill from the re-emerging West Nile virus in 2000, with a cluster of 14 patients from Staten Island. A few individuals from Brooklyn, and a woman in Manhattan also became sick. For the first time since the WNV arrived in North America, residents in New Jersey and Connecticut suffered from the clinical effects of the virus. All cases except the one in Connecticut occurred within a ten mile radius of one another, suggesting that infected mosquitoes from a common source (Staten Island?) might be responsible. Prevailing winds could easily distribute them that distance, and perhaps even farther, given the right conditions.

The weather patterns over the summer in the New York metropolitan area were quite different from those which occurred prior to and during the outbreak in 1999. In 2000, the months of June,

July, and August were rain filled, and were some of the wettest on record. Cool temperatures prevailed during most evenings, and some daytime temperatures were under 60^0 F; none exceeded 90^0 F. Despite this, many pools of infected mosquitoes and numerous species of dead birds continued to be discovered in many eastern seaboard states, including New Jersey, Rhode Island, and Maine. In addition, 65 horses became ill from the infection, and some died. The virus was clearly solidifying and expanding its position in the networks of wildlife in those states.

Over 450,000 people live on the 60 square miles of Staten Island, and thousands of them reside in single family houses located near large, standing bodies of freshwater, most of which are classified as wetland. Over the years, a constant stream of pollutants (acid deposition and particulates) exiting the smokestacks of hundreds of factories on Staten Island and from neighboring Elizabeth and Perth Amboy, New Jersey have produced severe degradation of all wetlands in whatever

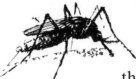

natural habitat remained in that densely populated region. Most of these former wildlife refuges have been affected to the point of elimination as functional ecosystems. Landfills on Staten Island also contribute heavily to the pollution of the last remnants of functional wetlands by leaching contaminants into their waters. All of these environmental abuses have combined to create ideal breeding conditions for *Culex pipiens* and other pollution-loving mosquito species.

Who Woulda Thunk It?

The re-emergence of WNV, this time in Staten Island, might have been predicted, based both on knowing the physical characteristics of the environment there, and the finding of large numbers of dead birds in the early summer throughout the communities of that borough. The hope was that the weather would win the day, suppressing the expansion of infected mosquito pools. Hope vanished with the news of the first case from Staten Island on August 4, and two more on August 12. An all-out ground-based spraying campaign began, but apparently with little effect, since new cases kept popping up on into the late summer.

Native wetlands were not the only sources of *C. pipiens*. Many residents of Staten Island have small ponds in their backyards in which they keep fish and aquatic ornamental plants. These artificial freshwater environments encourage the breeding of mosquitoes, and maintain a constant source of them even in times of drought. This situation is reminiscent of that found in northern Queens in 1999, when some abandoned backyard pools turned into sites for mosquito reproduction. No wonder then that the WNV entered human populations. In contrast, many other states reported similar large numbers of dead birds and positive mosquito pools, but without a single human case of WNV. Knowing where polluted, standing, freshwater exists is one of the important keys to understanding the spread of WNV, whether in Israel, Africa, or the United States.

Controlling Interests

Long-term control programs are what's needed most if we are to suffer minimally from the illness related to WNV. A thorough understanding of the breeding sites of the principal vector species becomes an essential ingredient in any effective control program. This means clean-up and maintenance of those sites in all areas where *C. pipiens* and its relatives normally breed, from a city's poorer neighborhoods to its up-scale properties, and from urban wildernesses to suburban backyard settings.

All sources of standing, warm, polluted, freshwater are suspect and should be eliminated whenever practical. When that is not possible, prudent use of larvacides is the next best approach. Spraying even relatively harmless (for us) insecticides from helicopters or trucks should be only viewed as a temporary measure not designed to offer anything but a momentary fix for a long-term problem. Environmental approaches have always proven to be best for maintaining control of mosquito populations, but they are initially expensive to implement and can be time consuming. However, as with almost everything else in our highly complex and modern world, the politics of any given situation may dictate more about what can be accomplished, rather than what really needs to be done. Ultimately, though, the choice is ours

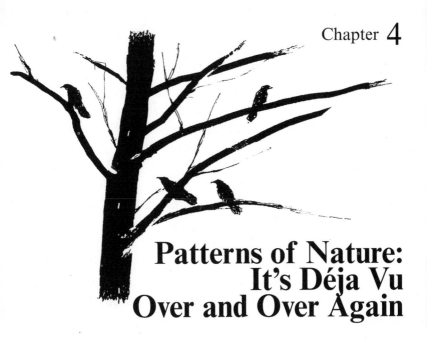

Chapter 4

Patterns of Nature:
It's Déja Vu
Over and Over Again

Brainer

The West Nile virus epidemic has now been described both from the human and bird side of things, but knowing what led to the outbreak lies in the details. What is viral encephalitis and how do we figure into its ecology?

To begin with, all encephalitis viruses can cause disease in humans and when they do, the membranes that surround the brain, and the brain itself, become inflamed and swollen. That's why we get headaches and sometimes become confused and disoriented. Fever almost always accompanies the infection. The disease can last for weeks, but it usually only affects us for a week to ten days. As we learned from the serological survey conducted in northern Queens by the CDC, most who are infected with the West Nile virus don't become ill, while a very small sub-set of individuals not only suffer from it, they can even die from it. When we recover, immunity is long-lasting, probably life-long.

All encephalitis-inducing viruses are related genetically, and are transmitted by arthropod vectors; insects (mosquitoes or biting midges) or arachnids (ticks or mites). The infection is almost never primary in humans for the simple reason that in nearly all cases we cannot maintain a high enough level of virus to enable any vector to acquire it from our blood stream.

The exceptions are notable in the flavivirus group. Two viruses related to WNV that cause yellow fever and dengue respectively, routinely allow transmission from person to vector to person. Birds or other animal reservoirs are not needed to sustain transmission. Unfortunately for us, the West Nile virus is also another of these exceptions. It can be spread from person to person via infected mosquitoes in some locales throughout the world without the need for introducing the virus each time by the migration of infected birds. These are endemic transmission zones for WNV. Typically though, birds in Africa and the Middle East serve as the disseminators of the WNV infection.

In regions of the world where good medical care is the norm, yellow fever and dengue fever make those who acquire it so sick that before the virus reaches high enough levels in them to enable a mosquito to become infected, they end up in the hospital. In rural settings, however, transmission of these two agents is from person to vector to person and goes on that way uninterrupted during an epidemic.

Out Of Africa

The key to understanding the conditions under which the WNV virus will or will not enter the human population requires a longer look at mosquitoes, climate, and birds. For the most part, human epidemics with WNV are sporadic in nature, making it hard to tell when the next one will occur. So what allows the epidemic to start, then gain momentum? And why does it always burn itself out? To answer these important questions about WNV, we have to delve into the history of the virus and the way it behaves in its native land.

There have been numerous epidemics of the West Nile virus occurring throughout the African continent, as well as in the Middle East (Israel, 1998, 2000), Europe (Italy, 1998; France, 1968, 2000; Czech Republic, 1997-1998; Romania, 1996, 1997), Russia (1999, 2000), and India. The disease in humans was first described in 1937 in a woman living in the West Nile district of Uganda. Her illness was initially mistaken for African sleeping sickness, a serious condition caused by *Trypanosoma brucei* (a protozoan) that is transmitted to humans and cattle by the bite of an infected tsetse fly. Later on, it was proven that she had instead been infected with a new viral agent.

This virus has a single strand of RNA as its genetic material, whereas all higher animals and plants have double strands of DNA as their hereditary molecules. According to Dr. Deubel, there are at least 23 known varieties (strains) of it, each one characterized by a slightly different sequence of its single stranded RNA molecule. In fact, the majority of these strains were characterized by Deubel and his group. The precise sequence of each strain's genome is equivalent to a human signature; no two are exactly the same, yet they all use the same letters, or in the case of the virus, the same nucleotide molecules.

None varies from all the others by more than 3-5% of their sequence, so the differences are small, but very significant. In any given outbreak, no matter where it may have occurred, all virus isolates are predominantly of the same strain, regardless of whether they were derived from humans or birds. That is why we can be almost certain that the strain of virus that infected the residents of New York City came from Israel and not some other place.

Walk Like An Egyptian

In Egypt, WNV exists as both an endemic disease (it causes disease throughout the year), and a sporadic epidemic disease (sometimes it causes disease, but not every year).

Egypt can be divided into two distinct ecological zones or regions. The northern shore and Nile delta defines one zone, and the southern Sahara desert the other. In the south, the virus is always entering the human population via the bites of C. pipiens. Even though it can infect all age groups, infection mainly takes place among the children. Transmission is year-round, and because young people are its primary victims, very few individuals suffer anything more than mild fever. Occasionally, a death does occur in this age group.

Transmission is mostly from person to vector to person, because children can tolerate quite high levels of circulating virus particles in their bloodstream without suffering much in the way of illness. Migrating birds are not thought to play a role here, but domestic fowl and mourning doves may serve as reservoirs for the virus, helping to maintain the virus in the local mosquito populations. Adults living in this southern zone, for the most part, are immune, since the great majority of them contracted the disease when they were young. As mentioned, immunity against the WNV is thought to be life-long. Therefore, few if any hospital cases and no deaths result from this pattern of year round, intermittent viral transmission in southern Egypt.

In the north, by contrast, the pattern of transmission is one of a sporadic epidemic, entering the human populations only rarely. This is due to a combination of climatic and ecological factors. To begin with, the weather is generally wetter and the climate is cooler. Since the virus replicates more slowly at lower temperatures in mosquitoes harboring the WNV, cooler temperatures reduce the chances for transmission to humans. Under these conditions, only birds seem to be susceptible.

Epidemics in this region are associated with West Nile-infected migratory birds that arrive in the hotter, dryer weather that predominates in late summer and early fall. A wide variety of birds native to Africa, carrying the virus, migrate out of their Middle European and Eurasian nesting grounds during late August, September, and into early October, on their way back to their winter homes. Along the way, they stop, feed, and rest in the countryside of Italy, France, Spain, Romania, the Baltic countries, and others, including the northern coastal regions of Egypt. When this occurs, it is possible for the virus to enter the local mosquito populations, fostering the initiation of an outbreak in humans.

It's a Bug's Life

Dry, hot weather is usual in the late summer and early fall, not just in northern Egypt, but all over Europe, as well. These conditions *force Culex* pipiens and its relatives into smaller habitats of polluted, warm, standing bodies of water. This invariably means they move closer to people, further increasing the likelihood that humans will be bitten. When the birds arrive, what few pockets of mosquitoes there are take advantage of the annual feast. Because the weather is normally hot when the birds arrive, the virus replicates at its maximum rate in the insects. Put another way, the mosquito is the "test tube" for the virus. As more and more blood meals are taken, the mosquito populations increase, and many of the newly hatched females have the virus, since it is transmitted "vertically" from the mother to her eggs. A mosquito is able to grow up in just two weeks under optimal conditions (warm, polluted water). When the birds leave, people are left to serve as the dominant food source for the now virus-laden insects. This is when the transmission to people may occur. Fewer birds mean more chances for mosquitoes to feed on and infect people. The onset of colder weather in the late fall lowers the reproductive rate for both the WNV in mosquitoes and the insects, themselves, significantly reducing the rate of transmission to people. The epidemic then slows down and eventually stops.

If the fall weather happens to be cooler than average, and somewhat wetter, then birds native to the area will still be around to absorb the increase in mosquito populations after the migrant species leave, and an epidemic in people is usually averted. Perhaps a few sporadic cases may result from unlucky encounters with an infected mosquito, as was the case in Staten Island, New Jersey, and Connecticut in the summer of 2000, but massive outbreaks are not the typical outcome under these conditions.

In the chronically drier regions of South Africa (the Kalahari desert), transmission of WNV is similar to that in southern Egypt and Israel; it occurs intermittently throughout the year. In contrast, along the southern coastline of that country, climatic conditions more closely resemble those found in northern Egypt.

For example, in 1974 a very large outbreak took place in Cape Province, located along the southwestern shore of South Africa, and involved more than 3,000 clinical cases and perhaps as many as 2-300,000 total infections. This massive epidemic reached its peak just after a deluge broke one of the driest, hottest months on record for that province. This arid coastal zone differs somewhat from the northern shores and Nile delta of Egypt in that it lacks a major estuary, but both areas tend to be dry and hot in the late summer and early fall. The drought forced the peridomestic vectors (those mosquito species that live next to densely populated human settlements) to fend for themselves within the boundaries of human habitation, initiating the epidemic.

In this instance, as in southern Egypt and throughout Israel, domestic fowl helped to maintain the virus year round in the local area. So when the heat and lack of precipitation drove away the indigenous wild birds, the mosquitoes turned to people and the abundant flocks of geese and ducks for blood meals. At first the rate of infection "smoldered," due to the limited breeding sites for the insect vectors.

The drought was broken by heavy rains, which supplied the virus-laden mosquitoes with new breeding opportunities, allowing them to expand their numbers in dramatic fashion.

This rain event helped to accelerate the spread of the virus to considerably larger numbers of people. Wetter conditions also attracted the wild birds back to their vacated habitats along the coast, and when they finally did return, the burgeoning population of mosquitoes returned to feeding on them instead of people. The epidemic in the human population then declined precipitously, and finally ended. The advent of cooler weather prevented any chance of the infection returning to the human population that year.

Because so many people were infected, even if conditions favored another outbreak in succeeding years, the likelihood of it occurring was small, considering that immunity to WNV is long-lasting. Immunity most certainly prevailed among the 300,000+ infected individuals, making another major outbreak in that region less likely in subsequent years, even though droughts may occur. This kind of infection pattern serves to protect the smaller numbers of people lucky enough to have avoided infection during the initial outbreak.

No Bargains In Those Basements

Bucharest, Romania experienced an outbreak of WNV in 1996 in which 527 cases resulted, and 40 died. Understanding the details of this epidemic will help to further define environmental conditions favoring the initiation of an epidemic of WNV. That year, the amount of precipitation for the summer was below average for the months of June-September.

While daytime temperatures were high, they were not significantly higher than in most other years. Nonetheless, the domestic mosquito population had to scramble to find a suitable source of water in which to breed. Migrating birds were not implicated as a major source of the virus, but a portion of the population in a variety of domestic fowl, including ducks, chickens, and geese, and several kinds of wild birds, tested positive for WNV. Lots of *Culex pipiens* and *C. molestus* mosquitoes also tested positive for the virus.

The confounding factor here was the lack of rainwater. How was the city of Bucharest maintaining its infected mosquitoes? Interestingly, construction of a new, extensive housing project, interspersed among the older city buildings caused a re-routing of city water into the plumbing of these new dwellings. Each had an open-ended sediment trap installed into its basement. A constant source of warm, polluted, standing water was now available for the mosquitoes. *C. pipiens* and *C. molestus* took full advantage of the new water resource and multiplied. The outbreak was over as soon as the weather turned cooler in October.

The French Connection

Sporadic outbreaks in Israel exhibit a pattern closely mirroring those that occur in southern Egypt and northern South Africa due to similarities in the ecological setting. Intermittent infections occur all year round.

The Negev Desert is a very arid, barren landscape, and military bases there attract what little wildlife there is. Outbreaks of WNV primarily involve soldiers on those bases. In other parts of Israel, goose farming has become a popular and highly successful commercial venture. Everyone knows that *foie gras* is treasured by the French, and Israeli goose farmers supply them with a large share of it. However, the drawback is that the geese become periodically infected with WNV when African birds migrate to that area on their way south. In addition, as in Romania, the geese are largely unaffected by the virus, and help maintain it year-round. Occasionally, a goose farm worker becomes infected. Mass killing of geese in attempts to rid these endemic areas of the WNV has been of little value, since migrating birds keep bringing it back to the region each fall. Transmission is usually higher in the summer and fall. The hotter the weather, the faster the growth of WNV and the higher the number of virus particles in each infected mosquito.

In 1999, an outbreak of WNV took place in southern Russia, in the desert valleys of the Volga River, and affected over 1,000 people with 40 deaths. Again, ideal conditions favoring the spread of WNV into human populations were in place prior to the outbreak: drought and hot temperatures.

In the summer months of 2000 in the south of France, in the Camargue region, many horses died as the result of their infection with the WNV. Transmission again was due to hot, dry weather, and limited breeding sites for Culex species concentrated the insects into the swampy areas of that region of southern France.

Roadside Diner

Why are North American native birds so susceptible to WNV, and why do crows, in particular, seem to be targeted so often? Other native birds, mostly songbirds (robins, blue jays, bluebirds, cowbirds) and raptors have also succumbed to the infection, but crows appear to have been selected for special treatment by the West Nile virus.

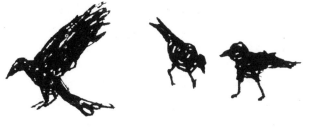

Crows are easily observed because they are peridomestic, highly social animals. They are much revered by native peoples in the American west, since these large black birds exhibit behaviors often attributed only to humans (cunning and guile). Crows have also occupied a place of respect in the world's folk literature (*The Twa Corbies*). This particular bird is often hunted but rarely eaten. The expression "eating crow" alludes to an all too familiar need to admit to failure at carrying out a given task that most of us have experienced at least once in our lives. Perhaps hunters of crows do not partake of their kill for fear of being placed into this pejorative catgory.

Crows are misunderstood probably because of all the noise a mob of them can make in the early morning hours when we want that extra half-hour of sleep on Saturday morning. Yet, the ecological services that crows perform for us in their daily routines are numerous. Crows consume huge quantities of pest insects and "police" the roadsides. They are routinely, and wrongly, accused of stealing seeds from newly planted fields (scavenging insects and worms uncovered by the plow is more their style), eating carrion, and of a host of other less-than-desirable behaviors. Usually, crows eat only the stomach contents of road kill and not the meat of the carcass. Surveys of internal parasites on crows verify this concept, and rarely turn up anything in the way of parasitic worms. Thus, they are one of the dominant species in our part of the world that helps keep the local landscape neat and tidy. Scarecrows of all dimensions and attire attempt to ward them off, but it's no wonder that none of them works very well, since these birds learn fast that these inanimate objects mean them no harm.

Crows are most often observed along the roadside in search of a meal. They relish the insects that hit car windshields and bounce into their marginal territory. If crows frequent the roadside even half as much as we think they do, then roadside ecotones (the edges of ecosystems) could be a major site of WNV transmission. The ever-present drainage ditches that border American highways can, and often do, function as breeding sites for mosquito species that require warm, stagnant, bodies of water. This is especially true for ditches that don't drain efficiently. Perhaps that is why crows are so often infected with the virus. Also, dead crows are easy to spot along the roadsides. This may account for the large proportion of crows among birds awaiting analysis in state heath facility freezers. Songbird deaths may be occurring at a similar pace, but many may be going unnoticed, especially if they take place in the deep woods where their bodies are likely to be scavenged by animals living there.

Perhaps even more relevant, at dusk, crows being the social creatures that they are, group into flocks of tens to hundreds. At night, small flocks join and form into larger groups called rookeries, and locate to the canopy of urban and suburban trees.

The sleeping birds, just by breathing in and out, create a constant stream of CO_2 that sinks to the ground and spreads out in all directions. Mosquitoes locate their prey largely by detecting the presence of this exhaled gas. *Culex pipiens* thus "rises" to the occasion. Flying low, they pick up the trail at the base of the rookery tree, and follow its concentration gradient up to the branches on which the resting birds are perched for the night. Dr. George Craig and his students at the University of Notre Dame in the mosquito biology division of the Biology Department conducted extensive observations on this phenomenon and were the first to report on it.

A recent laboratory-based series of experiments has revealed yet another way that the virus might be acquired by birds, especially crows. By keeping large numbers of uninfected crows in a spacious indoor cage, then releasing several infected crows into their midst, the virus soon affected all of them and they succumbed to the infection. No mosquitoes were needed for these infections. This indicates that WNV might be transmitted in the wild from animal to animal without an insect vector as the intermediary. This surprising finding raises new fundamental questions about the possible spread of WNV in wildlife throughout the eastern half of the United States, and more ominously, the remote chance that the virus might even be able to behave the same way in its transmission cycle to people.

The patterns of nature continue to fascinate and hold our attention. The spread of the WNV through the wildlife of North America has captured our interest, in part because of the extensive list of birds affected by it. Wildlife biologists will undoubtedly be kept busy over the next ten or so years assessing the damage and revising their predictions as to the overall effects of this infectious agent on ecological systems. Epidemiologists and clinicians will be doing similar studies on the human side of things. However, from the perspective of the virus, a host is just a host, regardless of whether it flies south for the winter on its own power, or takes the A train to a high-rise office complex in mid-town Manhattan. So goes the course of evolution.

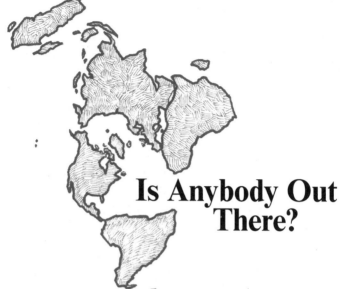

Chapter 5

Is Anybody Out There?

Misery Loves Company

James Taylor wrote a verse that summarizes: "The secret of life is enjoying the passage of time"; a reminder to all of us as to why we go forward each day with hope and expectations. Nonetheless, for a great number of people throughout the world, the enjoyment of life's pleasures is too often tempered by disruptions. Severe weather events, civil unrest, war, and all kinds of infectious diseases tend to dominate the human landscape. No wonder then that we frequently find ourselves out of synch with the trouble-free parts of our days and nights. Contemplating the larger questions of life—for example, our points of origin or ultimate destiny—requires extended periods of relative calm, which for most of us typically passes by as mere fleeting moments. It doesn't seem to matter much what line of work we're in, or where we live; Asia or the Americas, Europe or Africa, city or suburb, apartment or single family home. These intrusions pose threats to our very existence, and at the very least, divert us from the routines of daily life. So it was in New York City. Millions of unsuspecting people were distracted from their normal activities by the mosquito-borne West Nile virus. New to this side of the Atlantic, it has changed forever our view of the world we live in.

An unnerving event such as this represents the latest installment in a seemingly never-ending saga featuring a cast of the world's pathogenic organisms. The story of what happened that summer is not so much one about the outbreak as it is about the unknown world of microbial infections and how they can affect our lives in a moment. Fear of the unknown is what drives us to learn all we can about their sinister lives.

A Parasite Is Not A Person From Paris

Parasite is a term that constantly emerges and re-emerges throughout these WNV stories, so just exactly what are they, and why do we spend so much money, time, and energy trying to find out all we can about their lives? Because, simply put, they are always interested in ours. To begin with, most life on earth is of the free-living kind, interacting with each other, forming inter-linked dependencies that result in the establishment of contiguous ecosystems. Only a small part, the parasites, is devoted to living off the rest.

Parasites arise from a wide variety life forms. Numerous species of viruses and rickettsiae (bacteria-like organisms) are strictly parasitic. None of these can live without us. In contrast, most species of bacteria, fungi, single-celled organisms, worms, and six and eight legged animals are not parasitic. Just a few species of life forms in these latter groups have been selected to live off the resources we provide. Parasites are focused squarely on one job, to extract from us the things that are essential to their own existence, and they do so at our expense. To these specialized creatures, we represent an extremely successful biological system that has seemingly unlimited amounts of both food and shelter.

A House Divided

If a parasite needs a host to carry out its life, then what constitutes a host? Viewed from the parasite's perspective, we are the new house they have always dreamed of, located next to an upscale food market, and furnished with an intimate, spacious bedroom that offers the privacy they need in which to carry out their reproductive strategies.

It is indeed fortunate that most varieties of pathogenic disease-producing microbes are prevented from colonizing us by an extensive array of other microbial life forms already living on and in us. These user-friendly microbes are engaged in a wide range of mutually beneficial (symbiotic) activities, enabling us to go about unencumbered by disease. Our unseen companions help us digest food; make vitamin K, without which we could not clot our blood; aid in preventing tooth decay; and help keep our skin soft and disease-free. Most importantly, they keep out harmful life forms by out-competing them for the rent-free space we provide. Ecologically speaking, the human organism is actually a giant colony of numerous species (perhaps as many as one thousand) of invisible organisms that have, over an evolutionary time scale of some three million years, banded together to live as a single, integrated, highly mobile ecosystem.

Anyone who has ever been treated for cancer, or who has had to take large quanitites of antibiotics knows this. Eliminate the good ones, either by weakening our immune system with powerful chemotherapies, or by directly killing them off with massive doses of antibiotics, and the bad and the ugly are there waiting to move in. The lament, "There goes the neighborhood," takes on new meaning.

Who Wants To Be A Millionaire?

Life has been defined by some, obviously with a more pessimistic bent than Mr. Taylor, as a constant struggle for food and shelter. Certainly, this is the case when we contemplate the fate of our own microbial fauna and flora. The process of evolution continues to "invent" new organisms through the random shuffling of genes. Any new entity may strike it rich by chance and successfully colonize us. Establishment of infection is the microbial equivalent to winning the lottery's super jackpot. The World Health Organization recognizes at least 30 new agents that have emerged onto the human scene in just the last 20 years. This may seem like a big number, but when one considers the vast array of microbial species out there (perhaps in the hundreds of millions), we can consider ourselves lucky that only 30 have come to the fore, so far.

As the West Nile virus increases its host and geographic range in this part of the world, it will undoubtedly mutate to new strains that will become named after the places from which they were isolated, just like Lassa fever, Ebola fever, and Hanta-virus. In this way, the virus will settle into its new home and become just another fixture in the infectious disease landscape. In the meantime, we will have to get used to the idea. That's not a new concept for us, since, regrettably, polio, malaria, diphtheria, cholera, and Lyme disease are already household names.

For Every Action, There Is An Opposite And Equal Reaction

Why, then, haven't we lost out to this onslaught of parasitic organisms? The reason for this seems clear enough when we consider that the host-parasite relationship is not as one-sided in favor of the parasite as it may seem. We are, after all, blessed with an efficient immune system to counteract almost all attempts at colonization. It is composed of an interconnected, highly coordinated biological network of cellular and antibody-based defense systems that protect us from most harmful situations involving infectious agents and a wide variety of toxins. Throughout our own evolution, our immune capabilities have become refined by numerous encounters with microbes, so that today we are able to challenge and defeat nearly any and all comers. As a species, we have "won the day," even when many of those whose immune systems were not pre-programmed to fight potentially new disease agents died in the effort to resist.

While the human species does possess an impressive set of biological tools to ward off would-be invaders, the very young and the very old suffer more than the rest of us from encounters with pathogens, even if they do have the right genes. As we age, a general slowdown in information processing by our immune recognition system occurs, preventing us from reacting in a timely fashion to each newly encountered foreign microbe.

Infants have a different problem. They have to learn how to make an immune response by acquiring their normal share of viral and bacterial species from the surrounding environment. Coming into the world can be a genuinely painful experience, at least for the first few months after we're born.

United We Stand

In addition to our own biological defenses, we have created a community-based external system for the promotion of a disease-free life—public health. Good community-based health practices serve as a protective shield between us and pathogens. Public health is for the most part a silent partner. Most citizens who take advantage of its benefits are usually unaware of its many activities. Insuring a constant supply of safe drinking water, pathogen-free foods, a vigilant inspection system for slaughterhouses and for restaurant food safety, waste collection and disposal, and fluoride in water to prevent tooth decay are health-promoting services on which we have come to rely heavily as a first line of defense for prevention of illness. These accomplishments are modern miracles.

When a failure in public health services occurs, everyone within the boundaries of that service suffers. A good example of just such a breakdown occurred throughout the south side of Milwaukee in April 1994, when more than 400,000 people became ill within a three week period from a diarrhea-causing microbe (*Cryptosporidium parvum*). It had entered the drinking water because the south side's water filtration system was being serviced.

The time needed to replace the filters was only several days; time enough to do the job right without risk to the public, provided that nothing else confounded the situation. Unfortunately, a severe storm immediately preceded the outbreak, bringing with it an unusual warm spell, which combined to melt the foot or so of snow on the ground. The result was an unanticipated increase in runoff. All of these unrelated things came together and produced the ideal conditions for the outbreak. The result was a large influx of Cryptosporidium-laden runoff into Lake Michigan. Lake currents moved the silty water next to the intake pipes that Milwaukee uses to obtain its drinking water, and the organism became distributed throughout the taps of the entire south side of the city. North-siders were not at great risk since their filters were intact and not being serviced. It remains the largest diarrheal disease outbreak on record in the United States.

Considering that in the past we have had major epidemics of cholera and salmonella in this country, the Milwaukee experience reminds us that we still live close to nature, and that nature is still very unpredictable. In this case, it was human activity, coupled with unusual weather events. In principle, the West Nile virus story was not different.

Flea Markets

Several more examples will serve to reinforce our knowledge of the ways in which infections can spread among us. Plague is one of the better known diseases of humankind and has many general features in common with conditions favoring the West

Nile virus outbreak. It is caused by the bacterium *Yersinia pestis,* and is initially transmitted through the bite of the oriental rat flea, *Xenopsylla cheopis.* The flea serves as the vector for the bacteria, as does the mosquito for West Nile virus.

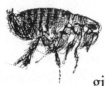

In the beginning of a plague epidemic, its ability to infect people is limited by the number of infected fleas and the number of dead rats in a given area. The fleas do not remain on a dead host. They lie in wait next to the dead rat anticipating the arrival of another host. The oriental rat flea would much rather bite a rat than a human. As long as there are enough rats for the fleas to feed on, no epidemics in humans occur. But when the number of rats diminishes significantly due to a rapid die off caused by the bacteria, and their preferred host is no longer around, the infected fleas turn to the next most available source for blood—namely us. But the flea has a problem. Its oral cavity (scientifically, it's termed the proventriculus) becomes plugged up with large numbers of the lethal bacteria that grew there from feeding on some of the ingested blood. Hungry for blood but not able to pump it past its congested mouth, the flea bites again and again, injecting the plague bacillus into victim after victim. Eventually, the flea dies of starvation, but in the meantime, it has initiated the infection in humans. This is not an efficient mechanism of transmission, and plague spreads slowly at first.

In the early phase of the infection in humans, bacteria locate to the lymph nodes and kill most of the cells there, causing the node to take on a blue-black color, hence the term, Black Death (bubonic plague). Once established in the human population, some become infected in their lungs, as well. When that happens plague can rapidly spread from person to person by droplet infection. This form is known as pneumonic plague. No fleas are needed. Therefore, one lesson we have learned from studying plague epidemics is that the same organism in the same host can present with two different patterns of disease. Early on in the epidemic, it follows one pattern, while later on, its pattern of spread is quite different.

When plague swept through Europe for the first time in 1348, millions (nearly half of the population) were felled in their tracks by this lethal microbial scythe. Yet millions more survived the Black Death, even though they, too, were exposed to the very same bacteria. Why? The most reasonable, biologically based hypothesis is that at least some of the survivors had inherited immune systems that were pre-adapted to resist. Those individuals unfortunate enough not to have been born of parents with this genetic background died upon exposure to the infection. This process is called "natural selection." Charles Darwin coined this term and felt that it most accurately defined the conditions under which a given species either survives or is eliminated by the competition. When Europe's population rebounded, the plague once again appeared, but this time far fewer died. Many of those new to the infection were descendants of those whose immune systems could do battle with this deadly pathogen.

The plague bacillus is also routinely transmitted to mammals in the United States by some domestic species of fleas, notably *Diamanus montanus* and *Nosophyllus fasciatus*. It is a common pathogen of squirrels and prairie dogs throughout the American southwest. Occasionally, unusual weather patterns alter the relative abundance of food for these two hosts, resulting in an increase in their populations.

When plague strikes in these over-crowded situations, sick and dying animals soon become abundant in and around human habitation. Some are captured by native American children and sold as "pets" to unsuspecting passing motorists. The animals eventually die, transferring their cache of infected fleas to the tourists.

In 1999, 18 cases of plague occurred in Arizona, fitting into this medical ecological description. Fortunately, all received adequate attention and their lives were saved, thus averting a potential epidemic. In 2000, thousands of prairie dogs died of plague throughout the western part of the United States.

There are other examples of atypical weather patterns and disease outbreaks that reinforce the need to pay attention to all of nature's signposts if we are to have any chance at all of predicting our own fates.

Isolation leads To Decimation

When the Spanish explorers arrived in the New World in the early 1500s, Mesoamerica went from a robust population of some 50 million, to fewer than five million in just over 200 years. The Spanish can take full credit for this dramatic decline in the native population, but it wasn't their guns that did most of the damage. Rather, it was their infections—small pox, influenza, and measles—that killed off the vast majority of those peoples. Today, Mesoamerica is one of the most densely populated places on earth. Its peoples have rebounded and then some, becoming part of a new global community. They share a gene pool for immune responses common with their European visitors through generations of intermarrage, and now have a biological awareness for most of the world's pathogens.

Ecosystem Services

Knowing that rats are the dominant host for the plague bacillus helps to focus attention on the fact that even in large metropolitan centers, other life besides our own goes on. In China, some years ago, the government deemed that sparrows were a pest, in part because they ate more than their fair share of the grains planted for harvest. An all-points-bulletin was issued to collect as many birds as possible. The program was a success. Unbeknownst to government officials, however, birds played a major role in preventing the transmission of certain encephalitis viruses by eating the adult mosquitoes that transmitted them. Removing millions of birds led to one of the worst encephalitis outbreaks in China's modern history. Bird control was stopped the next year, and the mosquito-borne virus infections waned

Many life forms, even those of which we are totally unaware, can be of direct value to us. This kind of activity is referred to as an ecosystem service. It also points up that we are all connected in one way or another, a fact we sometimes fail to appreciate until a disconnect has occurred. If the WNV continues to have its lethal effects on our native bird population, especially the raptors and those that eat pesky insect species, what will be the long-term effects for us in regard to the ecosystem services that they provide? By November 1999, 18 species of native birds had died of the WNV. By the fall of 2000, many more species had been added to that list, and in much greater numbers than in the previous year.

Is The Sky Really Falling?

Problems created by the introduction of infectious agents into naïve (unexposed) populations still exist. They remind us of the frailty of our existence, and go to the very heart of this book. Serious questions regarding our long-term chances for survival arise every time we contemplate such an event. How can we expect to co-exist with the invisible life all around us, that has the potential to do us harm, and evolves at a rate many times faster than we do?

A typical bacterium divides once every 20 minutes or so. Such a high rate of division should give us pause; any bacterial species has the potential to overrun the entire surface of the earth. This obviously has not and cannot happen for many reasons, including the fact that other microbes are competing for the same things—food and space. Antibiotics (penicillin, streptomycin, etc.) are produced, in the main, by soil microbes that secrete them as a means of carving out territory for themselves that can't be encroached upon by the competition. We have obviously benefited from this survival strategy by isolating many of those antibiotics and applying them to our own turf wars.

The act of division creates the opportunity for a mutation. The more individuals that arise from each division cycle, the more mutants there will be. For almost all life forms, including us, a single mutant is produced in about one in a million divisions. DNA is the double stranded thread that unites us all in this scheme, and it is at this level of replication that the mutation occurs. A mutant microbe represents a very small percentage of the total colony, but with such a fast replication cycle, even these small numbers can progress to large populations in a very short period. This is particularly true for viruses, which reproduce at many times the rate of most species of bacteria. Time is always on their side.

Divide And Conquer

Due to its relative abundance, mutant microbial life could find its way into our bodies and remain there. The influenza virus behaves exactly in this fashion, with new mutants arising continuously throughout the world. When they do, we are sometimes susceptible to infection, even if we have already had the flu or have taken the current vaccine against it. This is because a mutation in one of the proteins of its outer coat could have occurred. It is these proteins of the virus that our immune system recognize. Changing the antigenic composition of one or more of them means that we could catch it again. New flu vaccines include these changed virus proteins so that we can have a chance of avoiding the most serious pathological effects of the infection.

Another way the flu virus can change is by genetic re-assortment of its segmented genome among existing strains, without the need for mutation. This can occur when two or more strains of the virus enter the same host cell. Under these unusual conditions, a totally new antigenic strain of the virus, with characteristics of both the old strains, results. If the new virus happens to have a change in its surface molecules, then fatal epidemics occur, as was the case in 1918, 1957, and 1968. In 1918, nearly 20 million people died from this infection, alone. Because the flu virus is promiscuous, infecting pigs, ducks, geese, and humans, the chances for re-assortment is high.

International travel distributes new versions of this respiratory misery to all points of the globe. Today, The World Health Organization manages one of the most sophisticated monitoring networks for this single viral disease, with 82 member nations participating.

The West Nile virus is no exception to the way influenza behaves in human populations. It also exists as multiple strains, each being found in unique regions throughout Europe, the Middle East, Africa, and now the United States. In this case, however, re-assortment is not possible, because its genome exists as a single strand, whereas the flu virus genome is segmented.

Other examples of mutations with deadly consequences can be gleaned from the world of bacteria. The first ones of note to arise were syphilis (*Treponema pallidum*) and *Staphylococcus aureus*, a common pathogen encountered in many of the world's hospitals. Both of these organisms soon became resistant to penicillin, most likely due to over-use of that once powerful antibiotic. At first, resistance was slow to spread from the single source of the original mutation. However, in only 20 years (1960-1980), infections with these two organisms became increasingly more difficult to cure. Today, neither microbe responds well to penicillin or to any of its synthetic derivatives. This dilemma has occurred again and again, until now almost all other known pathogenic bacterial entities have evolved some strains that are resistant to nearly all known drugs.

Research scientists who study this phenomenon have come to understand the basic nature of the mutations that allow these "renegade" bacteria to live in the presence of most anti-microbial substances. Yet despite this important knowledge, preventing new mutants from occurring, or forcing them to revert to their former selves has not been possible.

Multiple drug-resistance in tuberculosis, HIV, malaria, and many other infectious agents has forced the international pharmaceutical industry to rethink its approach to preventing and curing infectious diseases. Vaccines are in, and antibiotic development programs are out. The few antibiotics that still work today, such as vancomycin and azithromycin, may not be as useful next month, and may be totally ineffective by next year or the year after that. It is only a matter of time; and remember, time is always on the side of the microbe.

We've Got You Surrounded

Will infections eventually force the human race to cave in and disappear like other species of extinct mammals? While infection undoubtedly has played a large role in tipping the ecological balance, especially in geographically isolated locations, it is unusual for a single microbial entity to cause the extinction of an entire species. We have been a growing population for the last several million years, and we continue to be, no matter what the odds, or so it seems. Have we just been lucky and avoided the inevitable infection that has the potential to kill each and every one of us? It seems highly unlikely due to the sheer number of us and the remarkable versatility of our immune system to recognize well over one million different permutations of foreign chemical structures. Perhaps we underestimate our biological resiliency. Nonetheless, it is still of utmost importance to find out all we can about a given microbe, or we will live or die at its mercy, and mercy is not a microbial concept.

First Contact

As already pointed out with the example of a plague epidemic, one crucial aspect of an infectious agent's MO (*modus operandi*) is the mechanism(s) by which it spreads from place to place. For newly emerging microbes, this is the toughest question to answer. We still do not know for example where Ebola virus comes from and how it enters the human population. Is it vector-borne, or droplet transmitted? Does it infect other animal species, as surely it must if it is to exist as a sporadic epidemic? If so, which animals and just how does it get from them to us?

If this one fact were known, then intervention to prevent it from spreading further would be possible. Acquiring that information is what is needed most if we are to stay ahead of the curve, regardless of the organism in question. In the case of the plague organism, knowing that fleas of a certain species transmit it to rats helps to define the problem. Controlling the rat population tends to control the flea population, as well. This approach has proven effective in the densely populated cities of India, where the rat is revered as a holy animal, but its role in disease transmission is also recognized. Rat control in India has probably resulted in the saving of hundreds of millions of lives.

Similarly, proving that only certain species of mosquitoes carry malaria and yellow fever allowed for the development of targeted control programs.

Taken to the next step, prevention of an outbreak of mosquito-borne illness is possible, based on knowledge of the actual numbers of mosquito larvae of a given species present in their aquatic habitats at any given time. This approach has resulted in the aborting of potential epidemics of malaria, encephalitis, and yellow fever by preemptively killing the insects before they hatch. There are many other examples which reinforce this basic concept of disease control.

As to the West Nile virus, medical entomologists and epidemiologists are still in the process of sorting out which mosquito species routinely transmits the virus from bird to bird, and which do the same from birds to humans and to other mammals. All that is known so far is that they are not the same mosquito species, and until we actually find out which ones do what to whom, targeted control programs aimed only at those species will not be possible.

A similar situation existed in the Americas with the yellow fever virus and its hosts: monkeys and humans. After intensive research that included experiments that resulted in the loss of human life, it was learned that one species of mosquito, *Haemogogus*, transmitted yellow fever primarily from monkey to monkey, while another, *Aedes aegypti*, transmitted it occasionally from monkeys to humans, and always from human to human. Both monkeys and humans die of yellow fever in this part of the world, since it was introduced here within the last 150 years. In Africa, where the yellow fever virus originated, the infection is transmitted in the canopy from monkey to monkey by one mosquito species, and to humans on the ground by another.

In contrast to yellow fever in the New World,

it never kills African monkeys, only people. Obviously, the immune systems of Old World monkeys have come into balance with this parasite, whereas we humans have not. This scenario is similar to the ways in which the WNV interacts with its own host species in those two geographic regions of the world.

Another critical area of interest to those concerned with containing the spread of infectious diseases is to define precisely the ecological conditions under which a given entity emerges onto the human scene. This has proven to be the most difficult area of research to carry out in the field. A part of this activity is referred to as "shoe leather" epidemiology because at some point during most outbreaks, it is necessary to conduct door-to-door surveys. Much has been learned about how epidemics start employing this straightforward approach.

Come Together, Right Now, Over Me

The initiation of an outbreak is dependent upon multiple factors, all of which must be present if the disease agent is to have a chance of spreading first from one individual to another, and then to larger and larger populations. The virulence of the infectious agent (how pathogenic and contagious it is for us), the mode of transmission (dispersal by sneezing and inhaling the infection-laden droplets, by injection of pathogens by a mosquito or tick), and our genetic pre-disposition for acquiring it, all play a role in the initiation process. Physical conditions often serve to enhance or diminish the overall success or failure of a given agent to rise to epidemic proportions, as in the scenarios for Cryptosporidium and plague outbreaks mentioned earlier. Unusual weather patterns (droughts, floods, hurricanes), air temperature, relative humidity, air currents, and human population density, contribute data that eventually must be fed into the general equation.

A few more examples follow that reinforce the concept that it's often short term patterns of weather that determine conditions under which a given pathogen succeeds or not in initiating an epidemic. Humans are exquisitely susceptible to the pathological effects of Hantavirus, whereas deer mice (*Peromyscus maniculatus*), the natural hosts for the virus, are not. In 1993, the deadly Hantavirus infected individuals in the Four Corners region of the American southwest, 20 of whom rapidly died of respiratory failure. The victims varied in age from ten years to 75 years, and none were related to each other.

The outbreak was triggered by unusually wet weather the previous year in that arid desert zone. Heavy rains stimulated rapid growth of plant life, and a subsequent bumper crop of pine cone seeds. Deer mice feed almost exclusively on pine seeds, and their populations in the wild soon rose to staggering numbers. The following year, the region experienced a more typical pattern of drought, leaving the burgeoning rodent population high and quite literally dry. They sought out food wherever they could, including the adobe houses of the Navajo. Mice excrete Hantavirus in their urine. So when more than three mice invaded a house, it sometimes resulted in a human infection. In 2000, 175 cases of Hantavirus occurred in the United States, with a 60% mortality rate.

A similar situation occurred in 1969 in Lassa, Nigeria. The multimammate rat (*Mastomys huberti*) invaded houses at the height of a drought due to an over-population of these rodents and a lack of an adequate food supply for them. Lassa virus is excreted in large amounts in the urine of this rodent species, as well. Infected rats carried the virus with them into the villages, urinating inside the houses, initiating a Lassa fever epidemic.

Predicting the occurrence of these two outbreaks before they actually happened was not possible at that time due to the lack of specific knowledge regarding the medical ecology of each entity. Today, we have a much better concept of the conditions that can lead to an outbreak since more have occurred. As the result, more warning can now be given to the public at risk by health officials should those conditions arise again.

W.H.O. Is On First

The general process of looking for trouble before it starts is called surveillance. Our immune systems do this day in and day out, looking for things that might hurt us and getting rid of them before they give us problems. Even single cancer cells that sometimes arise within us due to a mutation in our normal cell division cycle are almost always immune-eliminated by this highly evolved mechanism that seeks out cells that "look" different from us. Yet surprisingly, investing time, effort, and money into the development and maintenance of surveillance programs in our communities has often been given low priority in times of non-disease transmission.

"Forewarned is forearmed" espouses an approach to public health that has fallen out of favor in recent years. We live in a new millennium that caters to the electronically savant who move into hyper-space at the touch of a button on their digital imaging systems. Lest we find ourselves leaning in that direction, may we not forget how complacent to the new and unexpected we had become prior to the onset of the HIV epidemic of the early 1980s.

To prevent an epidemic due to an infectious disease from occurring in the first place, all the experts agree that surveillance is key. There is no substitute for it. Worldwide, there are many international agencies whose prime goal is to alert people to the next imminent danger from the natural world. The World Health Organization (W.H.O.) in Geneva, Switzerland leads the way, as does our own Centers for Disease Control and Prevention whose headquarters are in Atlanta, Georgia.

Founded in 1948, W.H.O. has become the centerpoint for international activities related to dissemination of information regarding all important diseases affecting the human condition. Malaria, cholera, tuberculosis, measles, influenza, and many exotic agents such as rinderpest, foot and mouth disease, anthrax, and a large number of viral-induced encephalitis infections are all being tracked by a carefully established world-wide reporting network of experts in many fields. Today, the W.H.O. is financially supported by 191 member nations. The agency has, for the most part, played a major role in the control and eradication of human suffering caused by infectious agents. Its vaccination programs have saved countless millions from the ravages of measles, small pox, polio, and influenza. It has linked itself together with The European Union, The United States Task Force on Emerging Communicable Diseases, and The US-Japan Common Agenda, forming a "network of networks."

The CDC has a local as well as an international

focus. Both organizations have an efficient red alert system in place to handle most emergencies. Between these two large bodies of experts, almost nothing of an infectious nature escapes into the human population without some warning. Add to that system the many departments of public heath for each state and city in the U.S.A., and we have adequate protection from almost all known agents. And there is the catch word: "known" disease agents. What about new ones that have yet to crawl out over the top of the microbial world's cauldron of genetic soup? How can we predict the emergence of something that has yet to happen? If we cannot, we must suffer the consequences. With some six billion of us now roaming the planet, we have the potential for an awful lot of suffering.

Spy In The Sky

Experience with well-known pathogens— malaria for example—can teach us a lot about future epidemics involving similar mosquito-borne pathogens, such as WNV. We can now access extensive information data bases about the spread of infectious diseases, the collection of which even ten years ago could not have been imagined. Technological breakthroughs have ushered in the advent of satellite-based remote sensing that reveal vegetation patterns, sometimes down to the species of plant present in a given ecological setting. Ground-based data collected in the field describing which pathogens and their vectors associate with which plant species, has led to the development of some remarkably detailed vector distribution maps based on pictures taken some 200 miles above the earth's surface.

Tropical parasitic diseases caused by malaria, leishmania, and schistosomes infect about two billion people, world-wide. Many of these unfortunate individuals harbor more than one of these life-threatening pathogens. All of these parasite species associate with specific vegetation types, and therefore are good candidates for yielding to detection by remote sensing.

Cholera is a well-known deadly bacterial disease, causing epidemics in humans, and epidemics are initiated when someone eats contaminated, raw shellfish. After that, spread of the cholera organism (*Vibrio cholerae*) is by fecal-oral contamination of food or drinking water. In nature, cholera performs an essential ecosystem service for some of the life forms living in the estuaries of the world. This activity has nothing to do with humans.

Blooms of single celled plants (phytoplankton), occur only at certain times of the year throughout the estuaries of the world, and are associated with subsequent blooms of a wide variety of microscopic animals (zooplankton). These tiny animals take advantage of the high population densities of the single-celled plants, and feed voraciously on them. The cholera bacteria help certain species of crustaceans in the zooplankton community to reproduce. By growing as a single layer on the entire outside of the two sacks that contain the eggs, these bacteria secrete an enzyme at just the right time to dissolve the outer shell of each sack. This allows the fully developed eggs and the bacteria to disperse into the water column. Repeating this cycle again and again allows cholera bacteria to achieve numbers high enough to eventually contaminate the filter feeding shellfish, which lie on the bottom.

The immediate practicality of remote sensing technologies is that it is useful in predicting where outbreaks of cholera will occur by studying satellite images of phytoplankton blooms in estuaries. The hope is that when unusual climatic conditions result in alterations of terrestrial vegetation patterns, these data can also be used to predict where new outbreaks of organisms, whose distribution is dependent upon them, will occur.

The Last Word (For Now)

The stories of the West Nile encephalitis virus outbreak in New York City touch on all aspects of a vector-borne infection, and because of that, it has attracted the attention of a large number of scientific specialists, not only in the United States, but around the world. Understanding its medical ecology through their good efforts is fertile ground for creating a new organizational paradigm for surveillance. Linking federal health agencies, state and city health departments, physicians and veterinarians, and research universities studying the environment, vectors and the diseases they carry strengthens the current configuration and form a worldwide network permanently on alert for the next wave of infectious disease entities. The internet will undoubtedly go a long way to facilitate this end.

Most scientists involved directly in the original outbreak agree that the WNV epidemic of 1999 has resulted in the establishment of lines of communications among groups that heretofore had never been in contact with one another. As suggested above, continuation of these interactions most likely will lead to a stronger surveillance system for all kinds of diseases, regardless of whether they affect mainly humans or wildlife.

But for New Yorkers, the West Nile virus outbreak represents just one more thing to worry about each day. In addition to the traffic and weather reports, the ball scores, and the volatility of the market, they now have to pay attention to mosquito spray alerts, become knowledgeable regarding insecticide toxicities, listen to the constant stream of new stories about dead crows and other birds, and wonder what the next spring will bring with it. Fortunately, these folk are a tougher than usual breed of city-dweller. Their past is studded with numerous transit strikes, a garbage strike or two, and several highly corrupt city governments. Undoubtedly, they will incorporate the West Nile virus as just one more strand in the rich tapestry of their daily lives, and most will go about living a reasonably normal existence in one of the world's great cultural centers. The world may never learn how the virus got into the Western Hemisphere, let alone into New York City. What is known for sure, however, is that the West Nile virus is here to stay.

People living along the eastern seaboard of the United States are now joined with all those who live in other regions of the world where the West Nile virus occurs, sharing their concerns and anxieties over this potentially deadly virus. It's remotely possible that the WNV outbreaks that occurred here may even have had a positive effect on how we now see ourselves as part of a larger global community.

Is anybody else out there? Make no mistake about this one. There most assuredly is.

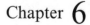

Chapter 6

Mosquitoes: Natural Born Killers

Running The Gauntlet

Throughout our evolution, there has never been a more real and present danger to our extinction than that which emanates from the bite of an infected female mosquito. Attacks by sabre toothed tigers, poisonous snakes, noxious insects, aggressive tribes of Neandertals, droughts, floods, famines, volcanic eruptions, earthquakes, and other such hazards of our earliest days on this planet pale by comparison to the destruction wreaked upon our species by infections delivered to our bloodstream through her dainty, hypodermic needle-like mouth parts.

Take the example of *Anopheles gambiae*, the world's most significant vector of malaria. That one species, alone, transmits a single parasitic organism that kills more than three million people throughout the world, more than two million in Africa, every year.

This means that in just the last century, more than 300 million people—more than the combined populations of Nigeria, Kenya, Egypt, and South Africa, or the entire population of the United States—have been felled by this one disease! If we could add up the total number of deaths from malaria that have occurred since our rise out of Africa some three million years ago, the figure would be even more staggering, and just as unimaginable. At present, a billion or so people at any one time are infected with it, making malaria one of the world's great scourges.

Since historical times, there have been writings alluding to malaria, but it was Hippocrates, around 400 B.C., who wrote specifically about the kinds of fevers induced by the four species now known to infect humans. The Romans, too, experienced the wrath of this protozoan infection, and actually named it; *malaria* means "bad air" in Latin. They believed the fevers were associated with the swamps and the foul-smelling odors emitted from them. Yet, for all of their accomplishments in the field of medicine, they had no idea that the disease was carried by mosquitoes. By simply building over wetlands and filling in stagnant bodies of water with construction projects—the building of the port of Ostia, for example—Roman engineers unwittingly became the first malaria control experts.

It was Ronald Ross, a young physician in the British Medical Service stationed in India in 1897, who finally made the connection between the parasite and its vector. He was working with canaries and Culex species of mosquitoes, but his findings quickly led the Italian scientists Amico Bignami and Giovanni Battista Grassi to search for the proper vector for humans. They eventually discovered that Anopheles species, exclusively, transmit it to us.

Thus began the modern era of vector biology, and the fledgling science eventually evolved into what we know today as medical entomology. Many other arthropod vectors were soon discovered: blackflies, kissing bugs, mites, ticks, sandflies, and biting midges. At the present time, the science of medical entomology is experiencing a true renaissance. The advent of molecular biology is leading the way into a future that promises safer and longer-lasting vector control strategies than the ones we now employ.

Other examples of mosquito-borne illnesses include the now familiar encephalitis viruses, of which the West Nile is but one, and some disfiguring tropical infections, such as elephantiasis (lymphatic filariasis).

A Fly In The Ointment

For many of us, it is the mosquitoes themselves, rather than the diseases they carry, that focus our attention on the concepts of vector-born diseases. Controlling arthropod-borne infections often involves containing the spread of the vector, and not necessarily the disease itself. To gain a deeper understanding for the connections between the West Nile virus and its hosts, it is to our advantage to know some of the intimate details of the lives of the vectors that transmit them to birds and to us. In that way, we can better appreciate how difficult it is to control their populations.

Mosquitoes are found world-wide, literally everywhere that fresh or brackish water exists. The only exception is the continent of Antarctica. This almost universal distribution pattern relates to the fact that they are really aquatic insects for most of their lives. The vast majority of species make use of natural habitats (swamps, streams, and sluggish rivers) in which to lay their eggs and to carry out their lives. Lakes and ponds offer breeding opportunities, as do brackish water tidal zones and estuaries. Snow melt in the tundra of the circumpolar regions encourages the production of huge, dense clouds of mosquitoes that often force caribou and other wildlife to seek refuge on the last vestiges of ice and snow to the north during the height of the summer months. Those animals not fortunate enough to make it beyond the range of the mosquito belt are literally sucked dry.

Couch Potatoes

Some mosquito species live peri-domestically, in other words, close to humans. They take advantage of small, aquatic environments that we provide by our own careless living habits. Discarded containers, abandoned wells, birdbaths, and backyard swimming pools that are not maintained properly can provide excellent breeding sites. They are found wherever we live, and only serve to further add to our discomfort when they are colonized by mosquitoes.

Eradication of these habitats presents major problems to city health officials in a sprawling metropolis like New York City. However, extensive experience with mosquito control programs in other cities throughout the world has taught us that cleaning up the environment is the only viable long-term solution to the control of peri-domestic species of mosquitoes. Getting rid of the garbage that accumulates between buildings and in empty lots, and maintaining an overall clean human habitat works. Spraying insecticides is, at best, temporary, and when applied improperly can do more harm than good.

Born In The USA

World-wide, there are almost 4,000 different species of mosquitoes, but only 150 or so varieties live within the U.S. They, and other two-winged flies, such as the common house fly, *Musca domestica,* are classified as dipterans (Latin for two wings). Most species of mosquitoes prefer to feed on animals other than humans. Nonetheless, each year in the United States, outbreaks of encephalitis remind us of the importance of paying attention to the ones that do feed on us, and the diseases they carry. Between 1964 and 1997 almost 8,000 cases were caused by a family of loosely related domestic encephalitis viruses (Eastern equine, Western equine, St. Louis, and LaCrosse). Many deaths resulted, including those from the West Nile virus.

Think Globally, Act Locally

Control and surveillance programs are the keys to effective public health-based control strategies aimed at reducing the numbers of vectors below the limits of transmission. In order to accomplish this daunting task, we need to know as much as we can about their biology. This adds up to gathering information on all those species that feed on us, as well as data on those that occasionally feed on us, but regularly feed on wildlife, such as birds. All in all, 150 biological stories need to be written. To make matters even more complicated, each species behaves uniquely in different locations, due to small, but significant, differences in temperature, rainfall, and the presence or absence of host species. Control thus becomes a local problem requiring unique solutions.

This Blood's For You

Why do mosquitoes need to suck our blood? It is used by the female insect as a high protein source, without which she could not produce eggs. The yolk of the egg is high in proteins, and these proteins are absolutely necessary for the embryo to develop into a larva once the fertilized ovum is laid on the surface of the water. The female chemically synthesizes egg proteins using whole human blood as the start-up material. Therefore, only the female needs to take in blood. Both the male and female mosquito feed on plant juices for their own nutritional needs.

The female adult mosquito has an exquisite set of tools for drilling into our skin, seeking out a capillary, injecting saliva that prevents our blood from clotting, and for sucking it up in a remarkably short period of time without our even noticing what is going on. The saliva of mosquitoes contains antico-agulants, anesthetics, vasodilators and lots of other substances that enable it to succeed. She detects our presence with special heat and odor-sensing organs designed with us in mind. Mosquitoes follow trails of carbon dioxide, which of course we give

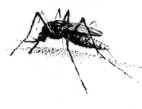 off every time we breathe out. When they get close, their heat-sensing organs take over and guide them to us, sort of like a heat-seeking missile, and potentially as dangerous.

By gently probing around for just the right spot with her sensitive palps, she inserts her hypostyle and enters the subcutaneous tissues. She then injects her pharmacologically active saliva, vasodilates a capillary, inserts the sharp end of her needle into the vessel, and pumps the blood into her stomach. The stomach rapidly fills up with the formed elements of the blood (red cells, white cells, and the like). At the same time she discards the liquid portion (plasma) through her anus. The equivalent process in modern medicine is known as plasmaphoresis, and is a method widely used by many blood banks to separate blood cells from plasma. Once the blood cell proteins are fully digested, which can take several days, the resulting amino acids are transported to the egg factory (the ovaries), where production begins.

Ova And Ova Again

It takes about two to three days for the female to make a batch of eggs, and she can produce anywhere from 30-300 of them, depending upon the species and the ambient temperature of the air. Since all insects are cold-blooded, at optimum temperatures (30-37° C or 86-98° F) they produce the maximum number of eggs. A lower temperature results in fewer eggs due to a lower rate of metabolism.

Once the eggs are deposited on water, several things can occur. In the genus Aedes, for example, the eggs are laid along the edges of temporary bodies of standing water, in containers of various sorts, and tree holes. The water level actually has to go down and give the eggs a period of time to dry out before they can hatch. The stimulus to hatch is supplied by the next rainfall, raising the water level above the eggs. The larvae emerge from their egg shells and grow, since there is now enough water to see them through their two week-long developmental cycle to adulthood before their environment dries out a second time.

In contrast, most other mosquito species lay their eggs directly on water, in which case they hatch as soon as embryonic development is complete. Again, however, larvae develop slower or faster depending upon the temperature.

There are four stages to a mosquito's life, and going though all of them is called complete metamorphosis. There is the egg, the larva, the pupa, and the adult. Larvae grow rapidly under ideal conditions, and each time they attain a certain size, they shed their outer skin (cuticle). They have four such periods of growth, culminating in the development of the pupa, known as the "tumbler," due to its rolling motion in water. The pupa lasts for about two days, after which the adult mosquito emerges. The whole cycle from egg to adult insect takes about two weeks under ideal conditions.

Larvae are called "wigglers" since they move in a herky-jerky fashion through the water. Because they need to breathe air, as they do not have gills like many other aquatic insects, they have evolved a specialized organ, the snorkel. It protrudes from their tails above the surface tension of the water and allows the larval insects to take in oxygen. When they begin feeding on planktonic organisms (microscopic plants and animals) and bacteria, the larvae wiggle down below the water's surface and filter feed through their mouths.

Some control strategies take advantage of the fact that the majority of mosquito larvae have to breathe this way. One effective method involves spreading an oily film on aquatic breeding sites, which clogs up the breathing apparatus and causes the larva to die.

Talkin' 'Bout My G-g-generation

Mating follows the emergence of the adult and this stimulates the female to take a blood meal, repeating the cycle. Female mosquitoes attempt to mate often, but are prevented from becoming inseminated after the first successful encounter with a male mosquito by a male-derived hormone delivered to her during the act of copulation. This unique aspect of their reproductive biology is shared by other insects, and control programs that take advantage of it have sometimes succeeded. The screw fly, for example, causes great damage to cattle when its larvae burrow into sites on an animal's hide that have been previously injured, perhaps by barbed wire, for example. Welts and sores soon develop and become infected. The hide is of little use afterwards. In some extreme cases, secondary infection, due to wounds caused by screw fly larvae, result in the death of cattle.

Female screw flies also can only be inseminated once. Releasing large numbers of artificially sterilized males into a screw fly breeding zone allows these altered males to mate with normal females, rendering the female sterile. The program has succeeded in Florida, and elsewhere in North America where this insect remains a pest of livestock.

Go Figure

An adult mosquito can live for about two weeks, but typically most live less than that. As the cold weather sets in, some species can "over-winter" as adults. Most species cannot, and therefore two weeks represents a very limited time in which to mate, feed three or four times, and produce multiple batches of eggs. Nearly 90% of all female mosquitoes fail to take even a single blood meal. They die without ever passing on their genes to the next generation. A few adults succeed for the rest, taking at least one blood meal and reproducing. Fewer yet manage to take two to five blood meals, and produce numerous rafts of eggs.

With malaria, it is this last small percentage of mosquitoes that efficiently transmits the parasite to us. This organism cannot be transmitted to the eggs of the insect. In other words, vertical transmission, such as is the norm for viral infections in these insects, is not possible. To give malaria to a person, it is necessary for the mosquito to bite at least twice; once to acquire it and the next time to deliver it to another person.

Lets consider the odds of this happening. To begin with, it takes the malaria parasite some nine to twelve days under optimum conditions to mature inside the mosquito. The insect only lives about one-and-a-half to two weeks at most in tropical climates. Very few adult female Anopheles mosquitoes are infected in any given endemic region of the tropics, even where the incidence of malaria can approach 100% at certain times of the year. To acquire malaria means that we must be bitten by one of these rare mosquitoes (about seven percent of the original population) that feed at least twice and carry the parasite.

These odds seem to argue against transmission, but the answer turns out to be a numbers game of sorts. The actual frequency at which an individual gets bitten each day at the height of the malaria season is staggering, sometimes exceeding one thousand bites a day. In a week or ten days in any endemic transmission zone, a person will undoubtedly have encountered an infectious mosquito and acquired the parasite. Transmission season can last several months in many tropical zones, and in some areas it is year-round. During these times, our actual chances of avoiding this parasite are somewhere between slim and none.

Know Thine Enemies

What about the vector species implicated in the transmission of West Nile encephalitis? What do we know about them? Can anything be done to reduce their numbers below the transmission limit for WNV

At least six different mosquitoes have been proven to carry and transmit the virus effectively: *Culex pipiens, Culex restuans, Aedes triseriatus, Aedes japonicus , Aedes vexans,* and *Aedes albopictus*. Recall that the virus replicates inside the female mosquito and infects her eggs, as well as infecting her salivary glands. Vertical transmission allows the virus to winter-over in adult mosquitoes. The next season, the infected females are ready to lay their clutch of eggs, which are also infected with the virus. In addition, they can take a second blood meal and transmit the virus to new hosts. The West Nile virus is known as a "promiscuous" agent in that it is not host-specific, infecting all kinds of birds, amphibians, and mammals.

One of the main factors in determining endemicity of WNV is the behavior of the virus in the mosquito, and this, in turn, is thought to be governed largely by climate and weather. Although this topic was already covered, it does not hurt to reemphasize the conditions under which it is believed that the virus is most likely to infect humans, now that the mosquito is the subject of our discussion.

In hot weather, the virus grows rapidly inside the insect cells and accumulates in large amounts in their salivary glands. The female can deliver enough virus to induce an infection in humans almost every time she bites. Under cooler conditions, however, the virus grows more slowly and may only achieve levels sufficient for birds to become infected.

This becomes an important consideration when we try to predict when the next outbreak may occur and where. Arid, hot climates, typical for most of the Middle East and many parts of Africa, have transmission all year round, while in temperate climates, sporadic epidemics are the norm, and seem mostly to occur in times of drought and heat. Since the northeastern United States is classified as a temperate climate zone, we would expect the virus to behave as it does in southern Europe. But so far, our experience is too limited with the WNV to predict accurately whether this is so. If 2000 is any indication, cool, wet weather does not favor outbreaks in people but does continue the epidemic in birds. Of course, as global climate changes affect the ambient air temperature patterns, where vectors are and how long they are able to reproduce will change. It could well be that *Culex pipiens* and its relatives will benefit from a warmer environment, prolonging the transmission season of WNV into the late fall and perhaps even making it a year-round worry for us all.

Culex pipiens

The habits of these five mosquito species is telling regarding the spread of WNV throughout the northeastern United States. *C. pipiens* is very common, with a worldwide pattern of distribution. Medical entomolgists believe that this species originated somewhere in Africa, then spread to the rest of the world. This may explain why it is such an effective vector for the WNV, since it we know that it, too, is of African origin. *C. pipiens* is a highly skilled stowaway, hitching rides on ships, planes, and railroad cars, and using whatever water there is in its local environment in which to breed. That accounts for it being found in nearly all major metropolitan areas. We now are aware more than ever, based on the 1999 experience with the dormant backyard pools of northern Queens, and the backyard bird baths and ponds on Staten Island in 2000, that it is an opportunist, and prefers to lay its eggs in stagnant, warm, polluted water. Sewage treatment plants offer some of the most luxurious accommodations for *C. pipiens*. An ideal companion for mankind, indeed.

Since *C. pipiens* feeds almost exclusively on birds when they are available, humans are usually safe from the diseases they carry. Nevertheless, they will reluctantly feed on humans when birds are not around. It seems that the biological imperative to reproduce overcomes any repulsion it may have for the taste of its next blood meal. Several generations are produced each year, and when fall approaches, the mated females of the batch preceding the cold weather over-winters inside storm sewers, and in other warm, protected sites. The next spring, they are ready to lay their eggs and begin life anew.

C. pipiens takes blood meals only at night, usually well after midnight, so roosting birds in trees are the perfect target. From our standpoint, its hard to acquire WNV by sitting out on the back porch and watching the sun set. We usually go inside afterwards, where there are screens on our doors and windows. There is little danger of being bitten by *C. pip-*

iens under these conditions. With a drought, however, this mosquito species flourishes, because of our sloppy habits with water. So, if the local native birds have moved on to greener pastures, *C. pipiens* females rely on us, exclusively, to survive and thrive.

Culex restuans

Culex restuans is a close relative to *C. pipiens* and is found in the same kinds of habitats. It feeds mostly on birds and occasionally on amphibians, but will also feed on humans if forced to do so. Because it almost never takes a blood meal from humans and its numbers are low, compared to *C. pipiens,* its importance to WNV lies in the fact that it may help extend the range of the virus into life forms other than birds. Eastern equine encephalitis has been isolated from a few mosquito pools of *C. restuans*.

Aedes triseriatus

This mosquito species lays its eggs in temporary bodies of water, such as tree holes, small containers, and the like. It can, depending upon the pattern of rain, have multiple generations each year. It is usually abundant during the summer months and prefers biting humans. It bites in the early afternoon, making it potentially a good vector for WNV, but most mosquito pools examined in all states reporting the presence of the virus have not implicated this variety as a frequent carrier.

Aedes vexans and Aedes japonicus

Aedes vexans and *Ae. japonicus* are two similar species that require temporary bodies of fresh or brackish water in which to lay their eggs. Like all Aedes species, a period of drying must accompany the process, and after a rainfall, the eggs are stimulated to hatch. *Ae. vexans* is native to the United States, while *Ae. japonicus* is a relatively new arrival to our shores, coming from Japan. *Ae. vexans* is considered one of the most significant and abundant pest mosquito species in New Jersey and surrounding areas. Like *Ae. triseriatus,* they are daytime (mostly in shady areas) and dusk biters, and actively seek out humans. They will bite birds on occasion. However, since people do not usually achieve high enough levels of virus to enable any species of mosquitoes to transmit it from person to person, their role in the WNV epidemic may be a minor one.

Late in the fall of 2000, *Aedes albopictus*, the Asian tiger mosquito, was identified as a carrier of WNV. This insect originated in Japan and was brought into the United States as a stowaway in tires shipped to Japan for re-treading. The eggs survived the return trip and hatched, eventually establishing thriving populations in many states. *Ae. albopictus* feeds predominantly on humans, so its potential as an important vector of WNV for us is real. Only time will tell as to its role in the spread of the virus, however.

Letusspray

Knowing all this information about our local mosquitoes might enable us to gain a leg up on their control, but it still requires a high degree of skill and determination on the part of mosquito control boards, as well as financial support to do so. Vector control programs exist in many parts of the United States, but those in California and New Jersey are among the best and most efficient, and deserve special mention. In New Jersey, the control board has functioned continuously since its founding in 1912. It originally arose from a need to reduce the population of Anopheles mosquitoes in order to help with the endemic malaria problem. Eastern equine encephalitis (EEE) is still considered a sporadic epidemic possibility in New Jersey and that virus keeps the control board on its toes. Pest mosquitoes also rank high on their list of public enemies. In fact, an oft quoted piece of humor states that the pesky salt marsh mosquito responsible for transmitting EEE is so big in size that it was once nominated for honored status as that state's bird.

The New Jersey Mosquito Control Board organization controls the populations of these five species of mosquitoes by a combination of targeted spraying and environmental intervention strategies. Draining polluted water habitats and maintaining the flow of local streams and rivers are its primary activities. When absolutely necessary, larvaciding and adulticiding is carried out, mostly around temporary bodies of standing water, with chemicals that rapidly break down, such as the pyrethroids. The board only employ insecticides at times corresponding to increasing larval populations. Aerial spraying for adults is usually not recommended, since in many cases, doing so is equivalent to trying to kill a house fly with a shotgun. Furthermore, as we have painfully learned from past experiences using chemicals such as DDT, chlordane, and the like, non-targeted spraying often adversely affects many species of useful insects, short-circuiting the ecosystem services they may provide to us.

Whether or not to intervene in the biology of a given mosquito species requires an intimate knowledge of its habits. Only then does it make sense to monitor its populations. Monitoring entails an extensive, highly trained work force that is ready to act at any moment. Low populations of larvae do not ordinarily require action. Ideally, when larval counts show signs of burgeoning, the control boards should spring into action.

In the absence of such organizations, establishing one from scratch is expensive, time-consuming, and demands the hiring of skilled personnel. Nonetheless, a full commitment to the control of mosquitoes using environmentally sound strategies with low health risks to us, such as the ones mentioned, is an absolute necessity. To do otherwise would be sheer public health irresponsibility in situations where mosquitoes figure centrally in the transmission of diseases that can seriously affect human populations.

Think Locally, Act Globally

Battles with mosquitoes continue around the world, and we almost always lose when we try and limit their spread by using chemicals. Many of the important species of malaria vectors are now immune to the effects of DDT and other powerful insecticides, and those that are not can still best be controlled by indoor residual usage rather than outdoor generic spraying.

Environmental changes that favor the destruction of the larvae work well, as the Romans discovered some time ago. Our own Tennessee Valley Authority was established primarily to control flooding, but it had a serendipitous effect in that it allowed for the development of a clever strategy for the eradication of malaria. Flooding by employing a series of high dams eliminated the swamps that lay along the banks of the Tennessee River. Mosquitoes were forced to use the lakes that formed behind each one for their breeding sites. Each lake level could be controlled by simply letting out water when needed. Lowering and raising the level of water at just the right time stranded countless millions of wigglers and tumblers on the shores. This practice led to the elimination of malaria, which allowed the opening up of that entire region to settlement and industry.

Today in Africa, the control of mosquito vectors is often hampered by political unrest and war. We live insulated lives here in our relatively peaceful, public health-conscious world. We don't get the sense that the problems of the third world are also ours. But the next time someone steps off an airplane from an endemic region harboring an infectious disease agent we don't have, but could, given the right conditions, we will think again about how important it is to think locally and act globally.

Chapter 7

Viruses Rule

"Great Fleas Have Little Fleas
Upon Their Backs To Bite 'Em
And Little Fleas Have Lesser Fleas,
And So Ad Infinitum." DeMorgan, 1915

To understand what a virus is and how the West Nile virus causes disease, we should first address a fundamental issue; namely what constitutes a life form. Unfortunately, there is no hard and fast definition. Science defines life rather loosely: anything is considered alive if it can replicate itself and then integrate into the lives of other living things, forming interactive associations. Since viruses are among the smallest things that can replicate, thereby increasing their numbers, are viruses alive? Well, this is somewhat of a trick question, since a virus particle cannot make it in the world by itself, but absolutely requires the help of another living entity, namely a cell. Without a cell to infect, the virus would not be able to carry out its replication cycle. Put into a microbiologically correct definition, all viruses are obligate parasites. One could argue, though, and correctly, that most parasites, large or small, need a host or they will perish. So, maybe a virus is just the smallest of all parasites; the lesser of all fleas, if you please.

We have already touched on the subject of parasitism, but only in general terms. If we start with one of our cells as a basic unit of life, then how does a virus compare to that? A mammalian cell, when placed into tissue culture under the right conditions, will grow and divide. Viruses cannot do that, no matter how enriched the growth medium is. Furthermore, a mammalian cell has many parts, all of which function to help it maintain itself in its environment. It is surrounded by a membrane that serves as a barrier to the outside, protecting the inner, delicate components from harmful things like too much salt, water, or even most infectious agents that try to enter it. The membrane is also remarkable in that it allows food, and just the right amount of water, salts, vitamins and other essential nutrients to enter, all at the discretion of the cell, depending upon its immediate needs.

Inside, it has all the biochemical machinery to make new structural components as they wear out or are used up during cell growth, and it manufactures all the enzymes it needs to catalyze its myriad chemical reactions. The cell can do all of this because of its extensive genome. By differentially activating its many thousands of genes encoded in its DNA molecules, all of its needs can be met. The genes are part of the DNA component of the cell, and it houses all of it in a special compartment, the nucleus. The mammalian cell is a true wonder. Imagine then, how complex an assembly of different cells we are. Humans are composed of some trillions of cells—thousands of different kinds—the great majority of which are in constant communication with each other.

Safe Cracking 101

What about the humble virus? There are untold numbers of different kinds out there, and most have only two components: a genome, be it DNA or RNA, and a very small house in which to keep it. The house, or more apropos, the cottage, is called a capsid, and consists of proteins all bound together in such a way as to completely surround the viruses' genome. Its DNA or RNA encodes for a few hundred genes at most, and then only in the very largest of viruses. The WNV has only enough genes to make more capsid proteins and its RNA genome molecule. So viruses are quite simple compared to our own cells. In fact, as mentioned, they are so simple that they are unable to grow by themselves. Some viruses may have extra membranes derived from the host that surround the capsid, but these kinds of infectious agents are rare in occurrence compared to the countless garden varieties that infect almost all free-living life forms on our planet.

Genetic Engineer, *Par Excellence*

Viruses are so successful, they have even been able to infect bacteria. These special viruses (bacteriophages) led the way for the molecular biology revolution when scientists realized that they could transfer small portions of the bacterial genome from one bacterial species to another using these viruses as the "shuttles." Viruses do this in nature all the time. It is one of the important ways that bacterial genes encoding resistance factors to antibiotics spread from a single mutant to other non-mutant bacteria. During their replication cycle inside the bacteria, the circular genome of the virus and the circular genome of the bacteria become linked together, forming one large circle. When the virus extracts its own genetic material after it finishes replicating, it often "steals" a bit of genome from its host cell, and during its next replication cycle, can give it to another bactrium. Many bacterial genomes show evidence for this exchange process. Thus, viruses are the world's premier molecular biologists. In natural settings, viruses help direct the flow of genes across species lines.

We have only recently learned that the oceans are full of different kinds of viruses, and that they most likely play an important role in the genomic exchanges that occur among algae, bacteria, and other microscopic forms of sea life.

Different Strokes

So, now we can see that there are major differences between a typical mammalian cell and an average virus particle. Perhaps we should redefine life to include organisms that are totally dependent upon other life forms in order to carry out their daily functions. This would allow us to place nearly all species of bacteria, protozoa, fungi, and all the higher forms of life into one list, and the viruses and rickettsiae (simpler, bacteria-like critters) into another.

The causative agent of bovine spongiform encephalitis (BSE), known as mad cow disease, derives from the replication of just a single protein molecule.

It is neither virus, bacteria nor protozoan. So BSE probably needs its own special place on the scale of living versus non-living things.

The saying: "successful systems attract parasites" is most apt, especially when we consider that many kinds of our cells (a very successful system of integrated molecules) have at one time or another harbored numerous varieties of viruses. We have all the necessary machinery that they need in order to make more virus particles. Since we are composed of thousands of different kinds of cells it stands to reason that there might also be as many different kinds of viruses out there which can infect them. Fortunately, this is not the case. Some viruses can infect almost any kind of cell (generalists), while others are specialized for life in only a few cell types. For example, the rabies virus mostly infects nervous tissue, and that is why it's such a deadly infection. Our immune defenses cannot easily counteract them once they reach a nerve. Should the virus eventually arrive at our brain, we invariably die. Herpes viruses are also "neurotropic," only we usually don't die from herpes. Others, like the Influenza virus, infect the epithelial cells of our respiratory tract. The West Nile virus, and all the other encephalitis viruses, too, home in on the tissues of the brain. There are viruses that attack the cells of the intestinal tract, and some that infect the uro-genital tract. Leukemia viruses live within our lymphocytes.

Breaking and Entering

When a virus particle attempts to "crack" our safe and enter a cell, it must do so in a fashion specific to that virus. The first step is called the attachment phase, and every virus has to do it. Attachment is usually dependent upon the presence of specific molecules on our cell surfaces. Without the ability to interact with the cell surface, nothing is possible for the virus. In the case of the influenza virus, a molecule called *hemagglutinin* on the virus surface is the molecule that interacts with our epithelial cell surface. Sialic acid is the receptor molecule located on our cell surfaces that interacts with it. In the laboratory using the tissue culture method, this virus can be prevented from attaching to lung cells simply by using an antibody made against the hemagglutinin molecule. Virus particles then cannot enter the cells, and they float freely in the tissue culture medium where they cause no harm to the cells.

A more subtle way to inhibit the virus from attaching to our cells would be to introduce sialic acid in high concentration into the test tube before putting the virus in with them. The hemagglutinin molecule of the virus would attach mostly to the free source of sialic acid, rendering the host cells virus-free. Each virus species has its own kind of host cell receptor molecule with which to interact. As researchers find out which ones are important, it will be possible to design and synthesize drugs that inhibit viral attachment molecules like the hemagglutinin protein, and prevent a wide variety of viruses from attacking us. Research on this aspect of viral biology is critical if we are to have any chance of fighting back against these fiendishly clever, infectious agents.

Alien

Once inside, the story varies, depending upon the type of virus. The single, positive stranded RNA viruses, of which the WNV is a member, have it the easiest. They merely un-coat their genome from the capsid (with the help of the host cell, of course), and soon after begin replication of its genome and the manufacture of new capsid proteins. The particle, with the genome inside, self-assembles, a truly amazing process. Under the electron microcsope, it's like watching a crystal form inside the cytoplasm of the host cell. As soon as the resources needed to make more virus particles are used up, the cell dies, and releases thousands of viral particles, which go on to infect new host cells. Eventually, the immune system catches on to what's going down and puts a stop to it. At that point, the patient starts to feel better. Immunity is long-lasting, often life-long.

Too Many Questions, Not Enough Answers

After all is said and done, the keys to understanding the ecological relationships that lead to outbreaks of the West Nile virus in human populations are two-fold. First, we must continue to monitor its ability to infect a wide variety of warm-blooded vertebrates and mosquitoes, and second, we have to further define and react accordingly to the patterns of weather that favor its transmission to us.

It has established a broad ecological network of infection and disease among birds, mammals, and arthropods that continues to widen even as these words are being read. How many species of birds will eventually be infected? What will be the effects of massive losses of native bird species due to WNV on other ecosystem functions and services? How many species of mosquitoes will serve as effective vectors for birds and humans? If we know which ones transmit it, can we control their numbers and reduce them below the threshold of transmission? How many people each year will become infected, regardless of what we do to stop transmission? Can the virus spread in human populations without the aid of mosquitoes, as it appears to be able to do among some bird species? Why does the virus only infect our brain tissue, and not some other, less sensitive tissue instead? Why do children suffer less, or not at all from it? How did it get here to begin with? Can we develop effective, safe vaccines against it for use in both horses and people? Where will the next epidemic occur in the United States? What are the climatic and weather patterns that encourage outbreaks of WNV in the United States?

We have known about WNV since 1937, yet during that time we have not made much progress towards fully answering any of these questions. Perhaps in the final analysis, the WNV epidemic of 1999 in New York City should be viewed as a new starting point for increasing our preparedness to deal with any mysterious strangers coming to our part of the world.

Epilogue:

Leftovers

The West Nile virus epidemic reminded us of what we already knew but had pushed onto the back burner of our busy lives; that is that we are all still connected with the rest of the natural world, subjected to the same rules as everything else that lives.

The unexpected events of that outbreak also elicited an instinctual, primordial fear of the unknown in many of us who had forgotten what it was like to be the victim of an infectious disease epidemic. Fortunately, only a few suffered from the virus, itself. The rest of us wondered if we were next on its hit list. Someone once said that humans are the only species that spends half its life worrying about things that will never happen. The rest of life on earth goes blithely about its daily routine largely unaware of any impending danger. But they, too, were at risk of dying from WNV, witness the number of dead horses, birds, and other animal species that resulted from just one summer's exposure to this newcomer.

Despite the fact that in 1999 only 62 people became ill and seven died, the WNV triggered a gut response in each and everyone of us who suffered through its long, slow ride through the neighborhoods of greater New York. That one event focused our attention on our own frailties as just one other life form on this planet. The fact that we have gone to the moon, nearly sequenced the human genome, and several times pushed the Dow over the 11,000 mark, does not negate the fact that we still must admit to our lack of control over our own environment. Indeed, we are not in control; it just looks that way when nothing catastrophic is happening.

In this affluent global culture, our taste for on-demand international travel, outrageously priced tall food, and rapid accumulations of personal income out-distance our perceptions of the real world. Exaggeration and non-real reality are in, real reality and truth are out. We have been culturally sucked into the Spielbergian glitz and seamless virtual world of DreamWorks-engineered *trompe l'oeil*. Heroes live 28 hour days and nights in the fast lane. Someone jumps off a building and lands feet first, unhurt on the roof of the next one some hundreds of yards away. Bullets stop in mid-air at the will of the protagonist.

West Nile virus in New York City represents a shoulder shaking jolt of nature's real reality. No matter how much we dislike that concept, it will not go away simply because we didn't invite it to the party. So we must now deal with it, and for a long time to come, so it seems. That we must find ways to deal with it which are compatible with our own lives is a given if we are to go into each day with a sense of place and peace of mind.

Literature Resources on the West Nile Virus

Origin of the 1999 WNV outbreak in New York City:

1. Lanciotti RS, Roehrig JT, Deubel V, Smith J, Parker M, Steele K, Crise B, VolpeKE, Crabtree MB, Scherret JH, hall RA, MacKenzie JS, Cropp CB, Panigrahy B, Ostlund E, Schmitt B, Malkinson M, Banet C, Weissman J, Komar N, Savage HM, Stone W, McNamara TS, Gubler DJ. 1999. Origin of the West Nile virus responsible for an outbreak of encephalitis in the northeastern United States. Science. Volume 286, pages 2333-2337.

Where WNV is found:

1. Smithburn KC., Hughes TP., Burke AW, and Paul JH. 1940. A neurotropic virus isolated from the blood of a native of Uganda. American Journal of Tropical Medicine and Hygiene; Volume 20, pages 471-492.

2. Melnick JL, Paul JR, Riodan JT, Barnett VH, Goldblum N, and Zabin E. 1951.Isolation from human sera in Egypt of a virus apparently identical to West Nile virus. Proceedings of the Society for Experimental Biology and Medicine. Volume 77, pages 661-665.

3. Taylor RM, Work TH, Hurlbut HS, and Rizk F. 1956. A study of the ecology of West Nile virus in Egypt. American Journal of Tropical Medicine and Hygiene. Volume 5, pages 579-620.

4. McIntosh BM, Jupp PG, Dos Santos I, Meenehan G. 1976. Epidemics of West Nile and Sinbis

viruses in South Africa with *Culex* (Culex) *univittatus* Theobald as the vector. South African Journal of Science. Volume 72, pages 295-300.

5. Katz, G, Rannon L, Nili, E. and Danon YL. 1989. West Nile Fever – Occurrence in a new endemic site in the Negev. Israeli Journal of Medical Science. Volume 25, pages 439-41.

6. Guenno BL, Bourgermouh A, Azzam T, and Bouakaz R. 1996. West Nile: a deadly virus? (Romania) The Lancet. Volume 348, pages 1315.

7. Han, L, Popovici F, Alexander, Jr. JP, Laurentai V, Tengelsen LA, Cernescu C, Gary, Jr. HE, Ion-Nedescu N, Campbell GL, and Tsai T. 1999. Risk factors for West Nile virus infection and meningoencephalitis, Romania 1996. The Journal of Infectious Diseases. Volume 179, pages 230-233.

8. Hubalek Z, Halouzka, J Juricova Z. 1998. First isolation of mosquito-borne West Nile virus in the Czeck Republic. Acta Virologica. Volume 42, pages 119-120.

9. Umrigar MD, Pavri KM. 1977. Comparative serological studies on Indian strains of West Nile virus isolated from different sources. Indian Journal of Medical Research. Volume 65, pages 603-612.

10. Lvov DK, Butenko AM, Gromashevsky VL, Larichev VP, Gaidamovich SY, Vyshemirsky OL, Zhukov AN, Lazorenko VV, Salko VN, Kovtunov AL, Galimzyanov KM, Platonov AE, Morozova TN, Khutoretskaya NV, Shishkina EO, and Skvortsova TM. 1999. Isolation of two strains of West Nile virus during an outbreak in southern Russia, 1999. Emerging Infectious Diseases.

Volume 6, pages 373-376.

11. Miller BR, Nasci RS, Godsey MS, Savage HM, Lutwama JJ, Lanciotti RS, Peters CJ. 2000. First field evidence for natural transmission of West Nile virus in *Culex univittatus* mosquitoes from Rift Valley province, Kenya. American Journal of Tropical Medicine and Hygiene. Volume 62, pages 240-246.

12. L'vov DK, Butenko AM, Gaidamovich SY, Larichev VF, Leshchinskaia EV, Zhukov AN, Lazorenko VV, Aliushin AM, Petrov VR, Trikhanov ST, Khutoretskaia NV, Whishkina EO, and Iashkov AB. 2000. Epidemic outbreak of meningitis and meninoencephalitis, caused by West Nile virus, in the Krasnodar territory and Volgograd region. 2000 Voprosy Virusologii. Volume 45, pages 37-38.

13. Cantile C. Di Guardo G. Eleni C. 2000. Clinical and neuropathological features of West Nile virus equine encephalomyelitis in Italy. Equine Veterinary Journal. Volume 32, pages 31-5.

14. Hubalek Z, and Halouzka J. 1999. West Nile fever – a reemerging mosquito-borne viral disease in Europe. Emerging Infectious Diseases. Volume 5, pages 643-650.

15. Lozano A, and Filipe AR. 1998. Antibodies against the West Nile virus and other arthropod-transmitted viruses in the Ebro Delta region (Spain). Revista Espanola de Salud Publica. Volume 72, pages 245-250.

16. Morvan J, Chin LH, Fontenille D, Rakotoarivony I, Coulanges P. 1991.Prevalence of antibodies to

West Nile virus in youngsters from 5-20 years old in Madagascar. Bulletin de la Societe de Pathologie Exotique. Volume 84, pages 225-234

17. Olaleye OD, Omilabu SA, Ilomechina EN, Fag bami AH. 1990. A survey for haemaggulination-inhibiting antibody to West Nile virus in human and animal sera in Nigeria. 1990. Comparative Immunology and Microbiology of Infectious Diseases. Volume 13, pages 35-39.

18. Panthier R, Hannoun C, Beyout D, and Mouchet J. 1968. Epidemiology of West Nile virus. Study of a center in Camargue. 3.-human diseases. Annales de L Istitut Pasteur. Volume 115, pages 435-445.

Clinical Information on WNV infection in humans and animals:

1. Asnis DS, Conetta R, Teixeira AA, Waldman G, and Sampson BA. 2000. The West Nile virus outbreak of 1999 in New York: the Flushing Hospital experience. Clinical Infectious Diseases. Volume 30, pages 413-418.

2. Sampson BA, Ambrosi C, Charlot A, Reiber K, Veress JF, and Armbrustmacher V. 2000. The pathology of human West Nile virus infection. Human Pathology. Volume 31, pages 527-531.

3. Han LL, Popovicic F, Alexander Jr. JP, Laurentia V, Tengelsen LA, Cernescu C, Gary Jr. HE, Ion-Nedescu N, Campbell GL, and Tsai TF. 1999. Risk factors for West Nile virus infection and meningoencephalitis, Romania, 1996. Journal of Infectious Diseases. Volume 179, pages 230-233.

4. Goldblum N, Sterk VV, and Paderski B. 1954. West

Nile fever. The clinical features of the disease and the isolation of the West Nile virus from the blood of nine human cases. American Journal of Tropical Medicine and Hygiene. Volume 59, pages 89-103.

5. Marberg, K, Goldblum N, Sterk VV, and Jasinska-Klingberg MA. 1956. The natural history of West Nile fever. 1. Clinical observations during an epidemic in Israel. American Journal of Tropical Medicine and Hygiene. Volume 64, pages 259-269.

6. Darwish MA, Feinsod FM, Scott RM, Ksiazek TG, Botros BA, Farrag IH, and el Said S. 1987. Arboviral causes of non-specific fever and myalgia in a fever hospital patient population in Cairo, Egypt. Transactions of the Royal Society of Tropical Medicine and Hygiene. Volume 81, pages 1001-1003.

7. Cantile C, DiGuardo G, Eleni C, and Arispici. 2000. Clinical and neuropathological features of West Nile virus equine encephalomyelitis in Italy. Equine Veterinary Journal. Volume 32, pages 31-35.

8. Steele KE, Linn MJ, Schoepp RJ, Komar N, Geisbert TW, Manduca RM, Calle PP, Raphel BL, Clippinger TL, Larsen T, Smith J, Laniciotti RS, Panella NA, and McNamara TS. 2000. Pathology of fatal West Nile virus infections in native and exotic birds during the 1999 outbreak in New York City, New York. Veterinary Pathology. Volume 37, pages 208-224.

Biology of WNV in mosquitoes and ticks:

1. Savage HM, Ceianu C, Nicolescu G, Karabatsos N., Laniciotti R, Vladimirescu A, Laiv L, Ungureanu A, Romanca C, and Tsai TF. 1999. Entomo-

logic and avian investigations of an epidemic of West Nile fever in Romania in 1996, with serologic and molecular characterization of a virus isolate from mosquitoes. American Journal of Tropical Medicine and Hygiene. Volume 61, pages 600-611.

2. Ilak MA, Mavale MS, Pransanna Y, Jacob PG, Geevarghese G, Banerjee K. 1997. Experimental studies on the vector potential of certain Culex species to West Nile virus. Indian Journal of Medical Research. Volume 106, pages 225-228.

3. Baqar S, Hayes CG, Murphy JR, and Watts DM. 1993. Vertical transmission of West Nile virus by Culex and Aedes species mosquitoes. American Journal of Tropical Medicine and Hygiene. Volume 48, pages 757-762.

4. Cornel AJ, Jupp PG, and Blackburn NK. 1993. Environmental temperature on the vector competence of *Culex univitatttus* (Diptera: Culicidae) for West Nile virus. Journal of Medical Entomology. Volume 30, pages 449-456.

5. Abbassy MM, Osman M, and Marzouk AS. 1993. West Nile virus (Flaviviridae: flavivirus) in experimentally infected Argas ticks (Acari: Argasidae). American Journal of Tropical Medicine and Hygiene. Volume 48, pages 726-737.

6. Reiter P. 1988. Weather, vector biology, and arboviral recrudescence. Monath, TP, ed. The Arboviruses: Epidemiology, and Ecology. Volume 1. Boca Raton, Florida: CRC Press. pages 245-255.

7. Barr AR. 1967. Occurrence and distribution of the *Culex pipiens* complex. Bulletin of the World Health Organization. Volume 37, pages 293-296.

The West Nile Virus:

1. Jia XY, Briese T, Jordan I, Rambaut A, Chi HC, Mackenzie JS, Hall RA, Scherret J, and Lipkin WI. 1999 Genetic analysis of West Nile New York encephalitis virus. Lancet. Volume 354, pages 1971-1972

2. Price WH, and O'Leary W. 1967. Geographic variation in the antigenic character of West Nile virus. American Journal of Epidemiology. Volume 85, pages 84-86.

Wildlife and WNV:

1. Rappole JH, Derrickson SR, and Hubalek Z. 2000. Migratory birds and spread of West Nile Virus in the western hemisphere. Emerging Infectious Diseases. Volume 6, pages 1-16.

2. Anderson JF, Andreadis TG, Vossbrinck CR, Tirrel S, Wakem EM, French RA, Garmendia AE, Van Kruingen HJ. 1999. Isolation of West Nile Virus from mosquiotes, crows, and a Cooper's hawk in Connecticut. Science. Volume 286, pages 2331-2333.

3. Work TH, Hurlbut HS, and Taylor RM. 1953. Isolation of West Nile virus from hooded crows and rock pigeons in the Nile delta. Proceedings of the Society for Experimental Biology and Medicine. Volume 84, pages 719-722.

4. Nir Y, Goldwasser R, Lasowski Y, and Avivi A. 1966. Isolation of arboviruses from wild birds in Israel. American Journal of Epidemiology. Volume 86, pages 372-378.

Current information on the distribution of WNV in the United States:

1. From the Centers for Diseases Control and Prevention. 2000. Update: West Nile virus activity-Northeastern United States, January-August 7, 2000. Morbidity and Mortality Weekly Report. Volume 49, pages 714-718.

Index:

A

C

Double whammy, 28
Dow, 11, 105
Drought(s), 10, 31, 43, 44, 45, 46, 47, 48
Ducks, 18, 47, 66

E

Earth quakes, 78
Eastern equine encephalitis virus (EEE), 30, 82, 93
Eating crow, 49
Ebola Fever, 57
Ecological network, 6, 7, 23, 51, 5254, 63, 69, 75
Ecological zone, 42, 45
Ecosystem Services, 63
Ecotones (definition), 50
Eggs (mosquito), 84, 85, 87, 90, 91, 92, 94
Egypt, 41, 42, 43, 44, 45
Elephantiasis (lymphatic filariasis), 80
Electron microscope, 21, 102
Elizabeth, New Jersey, 36
Emerging Infectious Diseases Laboratory, 7
Encephalitis, 1, 2, 4, 9, 19, 26, 30, 39, 40, 80, 93, 100
Encephalitis viruses, 2, 9, 22, 80, 82
Encroachment, 16
Endemic (definition), 42
English sparrow, 25
Epidemic (definition), 42
Epidemiologists, 9, 69, 73, 74
Epilogue: Leftovers, 104
Estuaries, 81
European trees, 28

G

H

Phragmites, 28
Phytoplankton, 75
Phytoplankton blooms, 75, 76
Pigeon, 29
Pigs, 28
Pine cone seeds, 71
Plague, 59, 60, 61, 62
Plague bacillus (see: *Yersinia pestis*), 60
Plasmaphoresis, 84
Pneumonic plague, 61
Poisonous snakes, 78
Polio, 57, 73
Ponds, 37
Positive stranded RNA viruses, 101
Prairie dogs, 62
Private pools, 13
ProMED (program for monitoring emerging diseases), 8
Promiscuous, 66
Protozoan, 79, 55
Proventriculus (oral cavity of a flea), 60
Public Health, 58, 72, 74, 94, 95
Pupa (mosquito), 85
Purple loosestrife, 28
Pyrethroids, 5, 6, 7, 93

R

Rabbits, 28
Rabies virus, 100
Rain, 11, 12, 23, 36, 46, 59, 71
Rain gauge, 11, 12
Rat control, 68

Also available from Apple Trees Productions:

Parasitic Diseases 4th Edition, 2000
Despommier, Gwadz, Hotez, and Knirsch